Vitrectomy

The journey ahead

Understanding a patient's mental state
during facedown and life's challenges
recovering from retinal detachment

Dicky D

FOREWORD

Dear Reader,

As I sit to write this foreword for the book, I honestly didn't know what to say more about or to say less to start with but my utmost intention in this book is to serve the purpose of making your journey as calm as possible prioritizing a good mental health if you are an eye patient or someone who knew somebody having Myopia, Glaucoma or a recent retinal detachment and had gone through intensive eye surgery. Here I talk about how my journey was as I am someone with myopia and glaucoma and in recent times had to go for a vitrectomy since I had a retinal detachment. I have been surviving life with vision in only one eye of left and a complete blackout on the right for more than decades and the recent retinal detachment and Vitrectomy have immensely invaded the course of my life

I am not a medical practitioner or an ophthalmologist. I wrote the book from the complete point of view of a patient and someone who had faced adversities concerning Retinal detachment, Vitrectomy, and the life after. However, one can easily extract information about the various eye problems through the internet or by Chat GPT, I doubt if it could tell a life experience that I had before and after the retinal detachment and its correction.

I tried sincerely not to bombard you with another blockbuster self-help or a guidebook. Consider this book like reading a story about a genuine man facing a bad episode in life and hoping to embrace life more strongly than ever. This book would greatly help the patient and the intending support personnel, family, and friends who want to gain insight and an understanding of the difficulties or challenges faced by such patients. but not making it a medical reference and technical medical book.

Happy reading

ACKNOWLEDGMENT

I want to give my sincere thanks to Som Bathla sir for his guidance in making this book a reality. His resourceful coaching method has helped me push forward to write this book.

 I would never be thankful and blessed enough to have my partner in crime, Nijara by my side during those gloomy hours of my life and take it with incredible willpower to arrange everything that was needed.

I would like to mention how lucky I am to have my lovely baby Thrishanayra, an inspiration for new life to be hopeful and pushed me to think ahead of that dark phase of my life. She is my all reason to be alive and stay motivated.

I will not forget the love and affection of my brother Mickey and his contribution to making my post-surgery recovery full of hope.

I would like to give my utmost respect and thanks to my parents for their unconditional love.

I would also like to mention my family and friends who supported me during those most needed hours of my life especially Dr, Mrinalini and her husband and my sister-in-law Chandini,

I still remember the nutritious and tasty food she cooked for me.

Last but not least the team of doctors of Sri Shanker Deva Nethra Laya particularly Dr. Manabjyoti Barman, Dr. Sahinur Tayab, and the entire staff of the OPD., I will always remain grateful to them.

Table of Contents

Everything was normal as it seemed on the surface, thanks to my ignorance, I didn't know if something like retinal detachment existed. Thanks once again to my ignorance, but I had to confront it and now am living with the consequences. It was certainly not an easy job, not for me and not for my family as well. My working ability has been hugely impacted after the Vitrectomy and has, to some extent, shattered my dreams and aspirations to ground. I was taking life as it was serving, with the ability to see with only one eye from the left. It was in the 9th grade I got to know about the complete blackout of my right eye; it was a blow to my parents as it was something unexpected. I had paid well for our negligence in medical education and health priorities. It was the late 90s, and nobody cared much about the internet revolution, at least not in the developing parts of India where I am from. At least I was not, nor were my parents.

More than a decade had gone and I was doing my regular job as a teacher in high school. Yes, I am blessed to get married to my loved one and have a baby girl, as she is now four years old.

I had a retinal detachment in my only working eye and had to go through a surgical procedure called Vitrectomy once and another two surgeries consecutively. It was quite hard and devastating to learn, except for the things as of now, because, for me, it was entirely new and has certainly changed the course of my life to a great extent. I have tried to capture the trivial thoughts and troublesome moments in this book. I have attempted to keep it as whatever I have been through and tried to keep it as it is from a patient's point of view.

 At times, I thought I was the only one.

This book will help those who are going through the same kind of gloomy situation and have the fear of losing vision and giving it all to come out as a winner, and keep that spirit alive in the wake of life.

"You are not the only one."

Retinal Detachment

Retinal detachment is a unique and serious eye problem that can cause permanent blindness if not treated immediately. This condition occurs when the retina, which is a layer of tissue that processes light, gets pulled away. If the retina of our eye gets torn, the fluid of the eye can leak from underneath and cause the retina to separate from the underlying tissue. People who have myopia or have an eye injury are prone to having the condition. Aging is also another significant condition to develop a retinal detachment. Other than that, people who have high levels of myopia in their eyes, have had cataract surgery, or have a family history of retinal detachment are also likely to have the condition.

Myopia

Myopia, commonly known as near-sightedness, is a refractive error of the eye that causes distant objects to appear blurry, while nearby objects remain clear. It is a common vision condition that affects a significant portion of the population.

In individuals with myopia, the eyeball is typically longer than normal or the cornea (the clear front part of the eye) has a steeper curvature. These structural abnormalities cause the incoming light to focus in front of the retina instead of directly on it, resulting in blurred vision when looking at objects in the distance.

Cataract

A cataract is a common eye condition that affects the clarity of the lens inside the eye. The lens, which is normally clear, becomes cloudy or opaque, leading to a gradual decrease in vision. Cataracts typically develop slowly over time and can occur in one or both eyes.

The eye's lens plays a crucial role in focusing light onto the retina, which sends visual signals to the brain. When a cataract forms, it interferes with the passage of light through the lens, resulting in blurred or hazy vision.

Glaucoma

Glaucoma is an eye condition that damages the optic nerve, which connects the eye to the brain. It is often characterized by increased intraocular pressure (pressure inside the eye), leading to progressive vision loss if left untreated. There are different types of glaucoma, but the most common form is called primary open-angle glaucoma.

The optic nerve is responsible for transmitting visual information from the retina to the brain. In glaucoma, increased intraocular pressure can cause compression and damage to the optic nerve fibers. Over time, this damage can lead to a loss of peripheral vision, which may progress to central vision loss if not managed properly.

I particularly mentioned the above last three eye conditions because they have affected my eye for years and most unluckily, I might not be only the one however, as usual, it is always suggestive to approach or get an appointment with an optometrist or medical practitioner to know more about your eye condition.

Chapter- one

THE WARNING

"Be like the cliff against which the waves continually break, but it stands firm and tames the fury of the water around it." Marcus Aurelius

Happiness is something that each of us wants to pursue in our lives, and it could be in multiple shapes; this paradox of happiness is endless in our lives. Perhaps happiness could be more beautiful and quite philosophical to write about, which could intrigue your heart, but I am about to talk about a disease, the alter enemy of happiness; it could have been much better to discuss the idealistic state of happiness than a retinal detachment. But here I am to tell how I felt when I heard retinal detachment for the first time. I already carry myopia and glaucoma; now this is some kind of shit tear in the retina, which we normally call a tear in the screen locally.

If you have picked this book, then you most likely want to know about Vitrectomy and retinal detachment rather than explore the various philosophies of the ideal state of happiness.

It was in the early spring of 2022, the time of the year when the leaves of the trees looked so new and everything was ready to embrace the newness. Could hear the practicing beats of the dhol, which is a kind of Indian version of drum, and the dancers danced out to celebrate spring as customary. which we in the state of Assam call this festive time "Bohag Bihu", and here I was waiting impatiently for the final report of the lab test, I was at one of the largest eye treatment facilities in the northeast of India. Sri Sankaradeva Nethralaya. The awaited moment didn't disappoint me much as I held the final report confirming a retinal tear. My wife was speechless as I was too; she could never have ever thought such a thing could exist, nor did I. The ophthalmologist called for immediate eye surgery, or else I could lose eye vision forever. It was an emergency call. We both sat quietly, trying to swallow our misery. After a while or more of the usual uncomfortable silence, I asked about the proximity of the success of retinal reattachment surgery. He simply replied that it was 90%. With a single surgery, this means that one in ten people might need more than a single surgery. So, "still there is the chance of a failure in the first attempt. It didn't boost my or my wife's spirit.

To the ophthalmologist's straightforwardness, he warns that if it's delayed, it may shut down the light of my only working eye permanently.

With a load of questions and heavy hearts, we both returned home, clueless about what we'd be served in the future, particularly me. She did her best to comfort me with her words to hold on to my worries, and I, with ease, pretended as if everything was normal. But from inside, I was anxious and super worried," the black clouds started to settle in my thoughts and mind." That's what I felt that moment. The date of the surgery was finalized since we were warned not to delay it. Back at home, though my wife tried not to be worried, she insisted on consulting her cousin, who is a medical officer at the GMC, Guwahati Medical College. We both were expecting some better proposition from her on it, and we were not disappointed. She instantly suggested consulting someone more senior in terms of having experience with treating people with retinal detachment and a good number of surgery experiences, cause in the medical profession the hands matter a lot. We didn't doubt her advice, and so the following day, we stepped into the cabin of Dr. Manabjyoti Barman. He already knew about the case and did some regular checks with the ophthalmoscope and asked us to consult the OT department to schedule the surgery date as soon as possible. He had a very tight schedule that week, which we got to know after inquiring at the surgery evaluation desk, and it was in an urgent situation that the surgery consultant talked with Mr. Barman, and he instructed him to put my name in the finalized date sheet of surgeries that week. It was his great endeavor and holistic approach

I was worried and anxious. My surgery was three days later. I was prescribed some pre-surgery eyedrops, and a day before or two, I had to get clear of the mandatory physical test.

That day after, my nights were never the usual ones, and I almost awakened that whole night thinking, Where did I go wrong? What had just happened? I had never asked for it. My thoughts were not in my hold anymore that night, and it was almost 5 am in the morning. I tried to shut down for a while, but it didn't happen. I decided to take the help of our most trusted "Google baba," and it didn't disappoint me as I got to know something more about retinal detachment and its treatments.

Notably, every disease shows one or more symptoms, most likely so it is the same with retinal detachment. The nightmarish symptoms most likely could be like: -

Symptoms and signs of retinal detachment:

Most likely, there's no pain associated with retinal detachment, but there are usually symptoms before the retina becomes detached. Primary symptoms include:

1. Blurred vision

2. Partial vision loss, which makes it seem as if a curtain has been pulled across your field of vision, with a dark shadowing effect

3. Sudden flashes of light that appear in one or both eyes

4. Suddenly see many floaters, which are small bits of debris that appear as black flecks or strings floating before your eye

These are terrible but the hard reality is that it does happen if the retina starts to detach. Before going further, I thought of putting a few more insights into those symptoms, particularly concerning floaters and debris.

Floaters are specks, dots, or cobweb-like shapes that appear in a person's field of vision. They may appear as dark or semi-transparent spots or threads and can move around when the eyes move. Floaters are tiny clumps of gel or cells within the vitreous, the gel-like substance that fills the inside of the eye.

Debris in the eyes refers to particles or substances that can float or be present in the eye, causing visual disturbances. This can include things like dust, eyelashes, or other small foreign bodies that enter the eye and temporarily obstruct the vision.

A few causes of eye floaters include:

1. Age: Floaters and debris in the eyes are more common as people age. The vitreous, a gel-like substance that fills the back of the eye, can change with age and develop clumps or strands that cast shadows on the retina, leading to the perception of floaters.

2. Diabetic retinopathy: Diabetes can damage the blood vessels that lead to the retina. When those vessels become damaged, the retina may not be able to interpret the images and light hitting it.

3. Near-sightedness: People who are nearsighted experience eye floaters more frequently. Vitreous syneresis also occurs at a faster pace in people who have nearsighted vision

4. Inflammation: Swelling and inflammation in the eye, often caused by infection, can cause eye floaters

5. Deposits: Crystal-like deposits may form in the vitreous and interfere with light passing from the front of the eye to the back.

6. Eye injury: If the eye is hit by an object or damaged during an accident, you may experience more eye floaters

7. Eye surgeries: Certain eye surgeries, such as cataract surgery or vitrectomy (removal of the vitreous gel), can cause floaters or debris to appear in the visual field as a side effect.

It is often assumed and seen that floaters start to appear after the age of 50, most likely. It's worth noting that while most floaters and debris are harmless and do not require treatment, the sudden onset of a significant number of floaters or flashes of light, accompanied by a change in vision, should be evaluated by an eye care professional.

I hardly can tell if it was by luck or bad luck that nothing like the above-mentioned symptoms, I faced in the given circumstances I was unaware and doubtful to remember any such symptoms occurred and I was too busy with life and hardly could notice any change in my vision except that I started to find it more than little hard to read the texts on my personal computer. I was skipping my dates of routine check-ups as well for the last three years. Along with all these, big planning was going on in my life, yeah, "probably bigger than my eye problem. "That's what I thought; otherwise I would not have been so careless about it. We were building a house to say goodbye to rented houses and apartments. It was exciting and some kind of a dream come true moments after four months as we step into our new house. It was in a matter of one or two weeks after we moved in our new house, I was at the eye care facility and everything seemed not in place. As the book "The Subtle Art of Not Giving a fuck" says that an old problem is replaced by a new, better problem, and at the moment, I didn't realize that, but felt pity for my condition and was feeling low. I wondered if I should have known about retinal detachment and its symptoms.

Chapter -two

I WAS BROKE

It is unsettling human nature that we often forget to feel grateful for what we have, but keep complaining about what we don't have. This cycle of complaints keeps on coming back after every new achievement, and most of the time, we feel broke and find ourselves detached from the factual reality. It is all right to feel broken; it is a kind of Defense mechanism of humans to respond to such a situation and navigate the facts of our existing life circumstances.

It was 21st May 2013, and a woman, along with her Sherpa was on an ambitious expedition to scale Mount Everest. when the Sherpa stopped and prevented her from stepping further, as their oxygen level was depleting and they were just about to scale the summit. The Sherpa hesitated to climb further; however, that woman with full determination moved further, and not to surprise the Sherpa didn't waste any time further and accompanied her without any complaint. After a struggle of two hours, they reached the summit victoriously. But what is so fascinating about it, Mount Everest has been scaled many times by incredible people from around the globe. What might draw our attention is that she became the first woman amputee to do it. Arunima Singha lost one of her legs while resisting some robbers on a running train, as she was thrown out of it, resulting in the amputation of one leg. In most such a given circumstances, one may lose sanity to some extent in accepting reality. So, in her case, too it was not unusual, but she miraculously replaced her grief with something more subtle and quite the opposite. She was determined to go through all the hardship that it takes to conquer Mount Everest because she didn't t want to be called handicapped and faced the sympathetic gesture of people around her calling her someone "Besari". She became a living example of strong determination and self-love and truly an inspiration for many to rise above adversities and fight back hard.

In the face of such adversity, when an individual is battling something unexpected, it is not uncommon to find oneself in distress and a stage of self-doubt and worry. The burden of an unclear future and inability to work due to the debilitating circumstances may leave one feeling heartbroken and overwhelmed. Along with all these, there is the financial situation as well, which possibly can amplify the burden. I had the same kind of feeling of grief and fear. I had to mentally prepare myself as well as my medical expenses. surely, I could have cut short my medical expenses if I could have approached another alternative like a government health center, but I didn't have that much time and confidence in government hospitals. It was not that the government health center didn't provide better treatment, but I doubted the lack of modern equipment and skilled hands. I might be wrong, but I decided to go on with the present circumstances. After all, I was not in a position to compromise because of the money situation, but on the contrary, it was as affordable as anybody could afford. I was diagnosed with a Rhegmatogenous retinal detachment and was prescribed a Vitrectomy. It was one of the other retinal detachments.

There are mainly three types of retinal detachments-

1. Rhegmatogenous Retinal Detachment: This is the most common type of retinal detachment and can occur when a tear or hole develops in the retina. The tear allows fluid to pass through and accumulate between the retina and the underlying layers, leading to detachment. Rhegmatogenous retinal detachment is often associated with aging, myopia (near-

sightedness), trauma to the eye, or previous eye surgery.

2. Tractional Retinal Detachment: Tractional detachment occurs when fibrous or scar tissue on the retina's surface pulls the retina away from the supportive layers. Conditions that can cause this type of detachment include proliferative diabetic retinopathy, where abnormal blood vessels form and cause scarring or a pockmark, as well as other disorders that lead to the growth of fibrous tissue on the retina.

3. Exudative (Serous) Retinal Detachment: Exudative detachment is caused by the accumulation of fluid beneath the retina without the presence of tears or holes. It can occur due to various factors such as leaking blood vessels, inflammation, tumors, or other health conditions. Exudative detachment is less common than the other types but can still result in retinal separation.

The most disrobing thought for me was the various risk factors that may affect the eye due to retinal detachments. My restlessness was at its peak, and no sooner had my worries started to take the form of frustration and depression as I was working with only one eyesight. The constant fear of losing my eyesight was there, lingering like the edge of a sharp blade. The overall thought was like a nightmare, and I had to survive it. The more

I thought about it, it saddened me, but I was confident with the medical team and my faith in God's will. I took the trusting help of YouTube and searched for the few available vitrectomy surgery video clips and some patients' experiences. Now by that time, my doubts about the surgery process were clear that it was not something like a cataract surgery but much more intense. But the scientific development in the medical sector and advanced technological aid made surgeries quite comfortable at least from a physical point of view. So, vitrectomy was a more advanced surgery. There is the elimination of pain and surgeries could be performed deliberately with ease. So, there were no worries perhaps about the technicality of the surgery.

Waiting for the day of surgery was quite heavy and more than dozens of questions were put into my thoughts. I was naïve looking for the answers and certainly not all were answered. I tried to put the broken pieces of my disheartened spirit into one and tried to reawaken my will to face the predicament of lying on a surgery table.

"How am I supposed to lie down on a table? It's hilarious", but technically it's called a table, though it had the functionality of a bed, amused me for a while but the many unsettling questions haunted me. I wanted to look for the better odds. I think it was quite normal for someone like me, who was about to get surgery, to fear a bit and face doubtful thoughts; that is why the medical counselling team or the surgery counsellor plays a handy role in smoothing out the situation. I realized that my predicament was not only a more physical one, but emotional and mental too. Supervision of an expert, self-assessment, and the help of family members and friends were the call of the hour.

Most likely, your family and friends will support you and will be along with you in that crucial journey, not unlike before, but I must say that the bottom line is positive words are magical and they can have an impressive impact on your thought process, but you are alone in your fight. You are the one who is about to lie down on that operating table. No one except you is going to understand your situation best but sometimes realizing it may take time. What I am trying to interpret is that self-dependency is the best way to handle the upcoming emotional turbulences because all the doubts and worries are meaningless till the surgery is done under the supervision of an expert and specialized team. To be honest, no one actually could accurately or precisely give a convincing road map of what it's gonna be like.

One thing I was certainly sure that my journey had begun, and there was no looking back.

A few questions that might create doubts could be:

What is the risk of retinal detachment repair?

Surgeries could always carry some side effects so is the same with retinal detachment repair. Though the process is safe and effective. The reaction to the various retinal repair surgery processes might vary from person to person and their previous health conditions. Reaction to general anesthesia might not be the same for all individual patients, particularly concerning breathing but it need not be a worry as the medical team will assist in all circumstances before and after the surgery. One thing that needs the most attention is that if the retina was damaged before reattachment, possibly there could be a permanent loss of vision. So, the bottom line is, that a retinal detachment cannot be left untreated without surgery most likely, and after surgery strictly need to follow the instructions and properly maintain it till the final follow-ups.

Infection- Retinal detachment surgery is not risk-free from an infection at the surgical site like any other surgical procedure. It will be well taken care of by the surgery team and the other medical facilitators to prevent any infection. Further taking care at home in a hygiene arrangement will lessen the risk of any infection.

Cataract formation – Retinal detachment surgery might increase the risk of developing cataracts. The timeline for developing cataracts after retinal detachment surgery is not fixed; it may take months or even years, considering the underlying health conditions.

Macular pucker- In some cases, scar tissue might develop in the central vision, which is macular, causing mild distortion or change in vision.

Loss of vision- Despite the best efforts of the surgeon, unluckily, retinal detachment surgery might not successfully restore vision or could possibly lose the vision.

Double vision- Technically termed as diplopia, occurs after retinal detachment surgery and might stay for two or more weeks and subsides eventually. In most rare cases, another surgery might be required to cope with the double vision issue if it stays longer than usual.

I dealt with the last two mentioned risks.

What can be expected in the long term?

Before concluding, what needs to be understood is that retinal detachment surgeries are complicated and sometimes need more than the best effort of the surgeon depending on the degree of the tear in the retina. Along with it the recovery takes time and does not always align with what was expected. There will be ups and downs but not always the same with all as my experience might not be similar to you or anybody else. To think about the expectation for the long term in the first surgery might be too early, I might sound brutal but this is what the harsh reality is, you might have the best result in no time but not all will have the same degree of outcomes. For an instant, the extent of vision improvement can vary from individual to individual. The main goal of retinal detachment surgery is to establish the retina and prevent it from further detachment. I have discussed it in more detail in the following chapter.

When is it too late for the surgery?

This question bothered me a lot during my initial days before the final surgery. I got to know that sometimes it's too late to perform the retina detachment surgery I mean retina gets back intact but it may not fully recover the quality of vision. But technically a lot depends on what part of the retina has detached. There is no such timeline after which it's too late for retinal detachment surgery. It is to be noted that if the macula or the central vision or the other vital parts of the retina have not gotten detached then the corrective surgery has the best probability of stopping the progression before the macula gets detached. If the macula has detached, technically it can be correctly reattached but the visual quality might not be the same as before. In general, the result of a successful retinal detachment surgery varies but detached macula and untreated retinal detachment exclusively affect the vision in most cases.

How long does it take to recover from retinal detachment surgery?

The recovery from retinal detachment surgery depends a lot on the type of detachments and the surgical method used. You might face some general complications after surgery as soon as the effect of the local anesthesia wears off, mild pain, redness, or other conditions might occur which leads to a delay in the recovery process. A person with a regular job and a family to feed might bother a little more about getting back to normal shit but being patient is the only key. A hell lot of our daily work depends on the equal execution of our eyesight along with our limbs so giving the required amount of duration to recover must be the foremost priority. If I have to give you a number then it might be like fifteen to twenty days at least along with the regular prescribed medication and other advice. In general, the same shit is considered that is the kind of corrective measures and the severity of the retinal detachment which is undoubtedly not questionable indeed.

The Key points-

☐   Recovery from a retinal detachment surgery depends on some factors like the type of retinal detachment and the corrective technique applied.

☐   Patience is the primary and crucial factor in recovering well.

☐   Generally, the recovery period ranges from 15 to 20 days at the very least.

☐   Following proper medication without fail.

Can Myopia [near-sightedness] increase the risk of a retinal detachment?

The answer is yes, Myopia or near-sightedness can lead to a retinal detachment. An article published in the National Library of Medicine dated May 13 2019, says that people with high

Myopia have the probable risk of developing a retinal detachment 5 or 6 times more than low Myopia. The article also illustrates the rising prevalence of Myopia globally particularly. among young adults from South Asian countries. Another website Advanceeyecarecenter.com points out too that a person with high Myopia has a chance of developing retinal detachment.

Can smoking increase the risk of retinal detachment?

Well, smoking is a crucial subject I guess to discuss because inhaling any kind of smoke is health hazardous but most of us still successfully get tempted by a cigarette. In This part of the world called India where I live, the government issued a long time ago to label every brand of a pack of cigarettes with a statutory health warning but it has not lessened its sales ever. Coming to the main topic does it increase the risk of retinal detachment? , yes it is. Smoking has been notorious for narrowing and damaging blood vessels resulting in a non-smoothing or compromised blood flow so in such a case the retina cannot be left alone untouched.

What are the chances of a second retinal detachment after a retinal detachment surgery?

The best answer might be given to you by your eye surgeon in this regard, however. a few things are to be noted. a proper recovery of a detached retina takes a good amount of time and even after regular check-ups and medication, there might be a need for another surgery. It cannot be determined in the first surgery itself. When I thought everything was getting good now, I had that unexpected blow, I was prescribed a second surgery.

How will be the vision after a Vitrectomy?

Vitrectomy is a complicated surgical procedure. It depends on the preference of the surgeon keeping in mind the type of Retinal detachment and other post-existing conditions. The recovery of vision after Vitrectomy will be slow, which means it might take more than a month or less to be able to recover full vision if silicon oil or gas bubble is used in the procedure. I have a complicated eye condition so my recovery periods and the pace were different. It almost took me one year to fully understand the amount of vision I am left with in my eye after the Vitrectomy.

What to be aware of before surgery for Retinal detachments?

Surgery always carries some risk. If you have general anesthesia, it can interfere with breathing. Some people have serious reactions to the medication.

If the retina was damaged due to external post-surgery factors before reattachment, there can be permanent loss of vision.

How a Retinal Detachment is repaired?

There are several types of surgery to repair a detached retina. A simple tear in the retina can be treated with freezing, called cryotherapy, or a laser procedure. Different types of retinal detachment may require different kinds of surgery and different levels of anesthesia. The type of procedure your doctor preferably performs will depend on the severity of retinal detachment.

One method of retinal detachment repair is "Pneumatic Retinopexy". In this procedure, a gas bubble is injected into the eye. The bubble presses against the detached retina and pushes it back into place. A laser or cryotherapy is then used to reattach the retina firmly into place. The gas bubble will dissolve in a few days. A pneumatic retinopexy can be done in an ophthalmologist's clinic.

In more severe tears, a procedure called a "Scleral Buckle" may be performed. During a scleral buckle, a doctor will place a flexible band around the eye to counteract the force that is pulling the retina out of place. The fluid behind the detached retina will be drained, and the retina should return to its normal place in the back of the eye. This procedure is done in a hospital, operating room, or surgery clinic. Local or general anesthesia will be used, and you may need to stay overnight in the hospital.

A "vitrectomy" is a procedure done for serious retinal detachments. It may require partially removing the vitreous fluid inside the eye. Local anesthesia is used and the procedure has to be done in a surgical facility.

What if there will be vision loss in some amount?

Vision loss would be least expected by the patient but Retinal Detachment is a complicated condition so the recovery process needs to be well observed and every change in vision has to be well monitored by the eye care team. If there is a loss of vision then one has to adjust to the new change. Life has to be managed without regret or heartbroken. A positive mindset has to be built under such unexpected circumstances. Low vision aids are to be prepared to manage basic things in life.

How will be life after a Retinal Detachment surgery?

In the worst scenario, one might have to be restricted from doing a few things in life. The vision of our eyes plays the most important role in whatever activity we do in life so, after an RD which is an eye vision-threatening condition, one may face unexpected outcomes even after a successful surgery depending on the type of Retinal detachment. One may have to make lifestyle adjustments.

It is most beneficial to be open-minded to discuss everything and sort it out with the surgeon and the medical team. Preparation of finance and post-recovery management should be well planned.

Chapter -three

The First Sign of Hope

Vitrectomy

On the day of my Vitrectomy surgery, I was acting bold outside but feeling numb inside, after all, it was the awaited day. As I was sitting in the waiting room, my wife was fulfilling the documentation and the other usual paper formalities, I was thinking hard about the surgery and was feeling nothing about it or about my position at that time. Maybe I was ready to board the bus of life's circumstances without question.

My silence was disturbed.

'Are you scared?' I asked my wife. "No", she replied, "are you?" I smiled and said nothing.

Later, I got to know that she was feeling heartbroken about this misfortune. I had nothing to say about it that time as well. It could have been much better if she had had another person walking with her that day, giving the genuine comfort that a heartbroken person deserves. I could understand how bold in actuality she was, carrying a heavy heart that day and waiting for me all by herself at the recovery hall with the other unknown faces around with bandages on their eyes, the scene was quite depressing.

I don't wonder how hard it takes for dear ones to make the adjustments to the occurring circumstances; I have witnessed it and certainly understood lately that it was a collective effort to get healed. Well, I am not trying to philosophies the predicament of such a situation, but it was no less than an instance of a drama that I never anticipated.

One of the nurses called out my name and asked me to get ready with a clean and almost new-looking set of clothes, which included a shirt, nice baggy pants, and a net-like something to cover the head, only the parts of the hair. The room was full of beds placed in alignment, which reminded me of the record cover of the famous' Pink Floyd', the name of which I didn't recall at that time. The bed was clean, and most of them were occupied by patients who were done with their respective surgeries. There was no chaos or rush-like situation, though people were moving and all seemed busy and obediently engaged with their responsibilities. I entered the changing room and here I was in full uniform, ready to enter the operating theatre, but my turn had not been called yet, so I had plenty of time to be there with my wife. At that point in time, I started to miss my baby girl.

She was with her grandmother and her uncle back at home. Maybe she was missing her father, too. For the last three years, I have been with her, mostly taking care of everything she needs. A full-time home-stayed father, and it had never been that I had not left her home with her grandmother before, but the day was not the usual one. Most of the earlier times and days was at home, which means my wife has a regular nine-to-five job, so I had to take the role of taking care of my baby girl and the household.

It felt as if I was not going to see her again, "Why is it so? What if I go permanently blind despite the surgery?". I asked myself inside my head.

The answer was simple: trust your surgeon and put your faith in the higher power. I had to gather my inner strength and be brave enough to face whatever I was served with. But the truth was, I decided to surrender myself to the flow of life and put my faith in the belief that everything would be all right.

I might sound sombre, but it was simply the way things were.

"Dicky Doley", called the nurse.

"Yes, I heard it." That's my name being called. So I was up for the operating theatre. A wheelchair was brought in, and an attendant was there to assist me till the entrance of the operating theatre. As the wheelchair rolled out with me sitting on it, I tried not to eye contact with my dear wife because I knew I wouldn't be able to stare at the hollowness in her eyes, the unsaid sadness she was trying to hide behind her constant, forcibly smile and so I was too struggling to calm that inexpressible sombre feeling.

We made the grand departure from the waiting hall to the fifth floor, where the operation unit was. I stood up from the wheelchair and made my way into the surgery unit towards the reception desk. One of the nurses took my check-in documents and instructed me to sanitize my palm and wait for further instructions.

I sat among the other patients waiting for my turn. One of them was pretty inpatients in waiting there patiently. He alarmed us as well that our surgeries would get delayed and cancelled.

"Everything in this country is fucked up, nobody cares, not even the nurses". He was whining.

It's customary to find someone who understands the seriousness of a serious situation no matter where you are dealing with agonizing waiting hours or minutes even seconds. It drains our limits of waiting to patience. Does it? At that moment it seemed to be true. I could say nothing about it but agreeing to him by bobbing my head when my test to wait patiently just might have started. There was certainly no way that a scheduled surgery would get called off for the day. That's what I thought.

As the clock ticked by, almost an hour or so later, the bench was left alone, sitting only me. Still waiting for my turn.

A kind and nice-looking lady nurse was sitting right in front of me. I didn't dare to break the uncomfortable silence that was hung in the air, but she did, and finally broke her silence about my peculiar-looking right eye.

 "How long has it been like that?" She inquired with genuine concern.

"As much as I remember, it's been like that since 1999". I replied.

 I was in ninth grade, then it didn't have the grey hue that it possesses now. It was one of the nights in the early fall of 1999, I was busy, most likely like my classmates, studying hard for the final board exam. I wondered why it was dark on the right but not on the left. I finally inquired about it to my father, he was in disbelief for some moments. He realised later that I no longer respond to a flashlight pointed towards my right eye, keeping the other eye shut with my palm. Next, the questionnaire started.

"Did you get hit by something in the eye today?" my father asked.

I replied simply, "No, my eye didn't get hit by anything at all today".

Confusion and concern enveloped everyone in my family that night

"Better let the eye specialist deal with that following morning. "My father concluded.

I genuinely don't recall how I felt that night and what was racing on in my thoughts. But I do remember that from that night on I transitioned into a person with the perspective of a single-eyed individual.

Once again, my name was called and this time, I was carried into the operating theatre. The air inside was much colder, probably because of the air conditioner. The surgery assistants were in full surgical outfits, preparing the surgery table for me.

I thought nothing as if I could see the perfect setups inside it, but I was not fully aware. That unexplainable fear was knocking on the door but I could not stop what was about to happen, perhaps for good only. I could see a familiar face approaching me as I lay on the operating table. He was preparing the anesthesia that was meant to be injected into my eyeball to numb the nervous system.

Injections in every shape and size can accelerate fear in our thoughts, and sp I was wondering how to react when it will be injected, and in no time the anesthetist started his work.

"Does it pain?", the anaesthetist asked.

"No", I replied. "Yes, it does sting a bit", but it is bearable".

He smiled, and I wished him good luck.

"Good luck, you too," he replied.

That's it, the Vitrectomy started.

Later on, Mr. Barman arrived and initiated the surgery. I wished him good luck, too, and so he smiled and spoke

"Everything will be fine."

I could not disbelieve his words. After all, words are powerful. I prayed in my thoughts for 'Vitrectomy' to be successful.

What is a Vitrectomy?

Vitrectomy is a surgery similar to pneumatic retinopexy, but is used for larger tears and usually needs to be performed in an outpatient surgery center. You'll be given anesthesia so you can sleep through the procedure. It is performed by:

1. A small incision will be made in the sclera of the eye.

2. A microscope will be inserted to see inside the eye.

3. Any abnormalities such as scar tissue, vitreous (gel-like fluid), or cataracts will be removed.

4. The retina will be put back in its place with a gas bubble.

5. Laser surgery or freezing will be done to repair any holes or tears.

6. In some cases, the surgeon prefers silicon oil to be inserted along with the gas bubble.

Severe pain is extremely rare after the procedure, but one may experience some discomfort. In some cases, you'll be able to go home that same day as long as someone else can drive you home. In other cases, you may have to stay overnight.

One'll need to wear an eye patch for a few days after the procedure to make sure the eye heals completely.

The eyelid speculum was put in to be operated eye. I could feel nothing but I could see an array of lights that were appearing and disappearing at the same moment. It seemed as if my eye was blocked by a cast of yellow light. I was temporarily blind I could say was of that moment but I could hear everything that was happening around me. As I had earlier visited the various available video contents on Vitrectomy on YouTube, I could now imagine precisely the steps the surgeon was about to take.

What a loser am I? – I should be operating my own eye now if I could know the steps so precisely by watching YouTube videos. But the bottom line is I was trying to be hopeful, I didn't want to be hopeless in my thoughts while lying on the operation table and maybe my imagination at those moments was an initiation of being hopeful and without fear and keeping control of my thoughts.

It's an old saying that" If you don't look out for your own well-being then no one will". It is our own determination to heal that does 50% of our healing or sometimes more than that.

Physiological and psychological stress before and during surgery might accelerate the rise in blood pressure but a lot more depends on the previous fitness of the patient and the strict monitoring of the surgery team. I didn't want to spoil the moments, and I couldn't help but entertain a bit of dark humour to cope with my fears. I would say with a sarcastic tone, but I was scared, what if the surgical gamble went in vain? I was trying from my side as well to make it to the finish line without any other complications. I didn't know how to react in the gloomy and sterile operating room while a Vitrectomy was going on. Perhaps it was normal to be plagued with worries like that during such an intensive procedure. After some moments that I didn't know, I started to think about my baby girl, my loving wife, and my dear ones, I felt an urge to release it all through tears. it was not my turn not yet, but I felt like that if it was my last. The constant fear of not being able to see the face of my baby girl again kept on coming but in no time the surgery of Vitrectomy drew to a close and the final words of the Doctor provided a lifeline back to reality.

"It's done, it's done quite well "

I released my breath if I was holding it for very long and was happy that I made it but,

"Yeah! There's always a "but" that might appear most of the time".

I was blackout, not the kind that comes from being knocked out, but I was plunged into complete blindness. I could see only darkness, a complete pitch black. I could see nothing by one eye being operated and wrapped in bandage and protected with an eye shield, and the other being blind permanently I was sensing more deeply to navigate my surroundings as I was guided by the surgery assistants to step down from the operation table to my left cause the portable stairs were positioned on the left side, I clung to their supporting arms as they carefully guided me till I reached the wheelchair safely that was meant to escort me out of the operating room to the observation area where I could be monitored.

Here I was once again testing the complete blackout I would say and as I was escorted out of the operation theatre, I could also feel that goosebump that I could hit myself on something as if it may hit my head or feet though I was sitting on a wheelchair and the ward boy was careful of not even any bump could hit the wheelchair hard. I could feel that, though I can't see it technically. No sooner was I here at the monitoring room, or what to call it? a waiting room, but what best described that room could be my salvation room from this uncomfortable darkness. I was asked by the ward boy to stand up from the wheelchair and reach out on my own to the bed on my right.

" I couldn't believe it, that's how a blind person should be treated?" I complained to myself.

I hesitated and held myself back from leaving the Wheelchair. I wasn't sure and at that, I heard my wife's voice and could feel her hands on my arms, ready to guide me up from that loyal service full Wheelchair to my bed.

"Step out to your right", she instructed. The ward boy too nodded, "To your right, sir, step out slowly and just reach out your hand, you will get the bed".

The bed was right there, he was not lying, and I managed myself up to the bed with full help from my wife. Now I could feel the soft, tender mattress and the supportive pillow to rest my head on. As I was lying comfortably in the bed, I still could sense the hustle that the room was filled with.

I asked my wife, "Is it the same bed I was in this morning before the surgery?"

"No that's a different one and we are in a different room section too", she answered.

So all the beds are full I guessed and was wondering if the pain starts, how long and painful it could be?

"Okay pain is inevitable, it is not going to stay forever, I knew that line and sincerely believed it but the real worry started now. Yeah! more practical kind of."

As of now, I was in Annastacia which will slowly fade away and I knew that it will hit me very hard. Leaving that worry aside for a while, me and my wife were both clueless about our next step.

Caution- proper planning is a must for any medical condition or surgery depending on your present circumstances and your financial Accountability.

It is obvious that we would stay in the hospital that evening but to our dismay, it was informed that we had to leave not as soon as possible but right after we consulted with the chief nurse there. Who would provide all the necessary and mandatory post-surgery medication and the next check-up schedule?

"Now what?", I murmured, and that agony circumstance was teaching me as if I was a grade A newcomer," yeah your teacher going to welcome you and get you your new friend in the school" but, not in my case. That stubborn fate was pointing at me and asking, how's going, bro? "I would sue you in the court" that's what I thought to reply back.

Instead, my wife replied, "If so then we would stay in the nearest hotel or guest house, probably there would be some near such a big eye care center".

Probably you might be wondering that in surgery cases usually the patients stay in the facility so why not me? It depends on the degree of surgery that was done and most likely in my case, I was comparing Vitrectomy would be like normal cataract surgery and the surgery might have been done within one hour to maximum but, it took nearly three hours till I was moved from the surgery facility to the post-surgery monitoring room.

The time came when my name was called once again by the nurse who was counseling all the other patients before they left the room. With gentle precision, she outlined the meticulous regime I needed to follow until the next day when my eye would be relieved from the bandage. A thorough check-up awaited the next day.

'thank you, 'I replied, though I could see no one.

Once again, the trusted wheelchair was summoned, and obediently, I was escorted to the ground floor and I could feel my wife walking beside the wheelchair. She booked an Uber all ready to take us to our next destination- 'my sister-in-law's apartment'.

While we were astounded to know from one of the attendants that we had to leave after more than an hour. So, we had to decide on where to stay the night out since we could not get back to our home at the hilltop.

'Yes, we had a plot of land and our home in a hilly area in the city where the roadways are not that good, I mean not commutable even in a car prior to my condition'.

I will not detail much about my locality cause I think every place has its own unique attributes whether you might like it or dislike it.

The Uber Wala pulled up and I was carefully guided by two assistants from the hospital who helped me to get into the backseat, mindful of my delicate condition.

Despite the instinct to recline like any passenger would have done, I had to adhere to a new directive: The head down position, yes, a new way of positioning my body till I was healed. It's the 'head-down posture' that I had to retain for the next month or longer. No matter what I might do I had to keep my head downward. At that moment, I could not foresee the difficulty level that I would face in the coming days as I was sitting behind, maintaining the exact position I had just said. Tell you what, I could feel the beam of light thrown by the cars on the road and it triggered a surreal feeling if my eyeball was dancing up and down and felt like a very squeezy thing like slime whenever the car hits a jolt and bump on the road.

'Don't worry the Uber driver was very cautiously driving through the Indian roads, he knew about my delicate condition so he was careful too'.

I could feel the same array of familiar traffic sounds and the hustle that was going on from the back seat. I had imagined it to be perfectly the way I thought at that time. I was going through a kind of feeling inexpressible only could feel that a blind person might feel the same way. It was a complete blackout technically.

The car stopped and the door was opened. I was not surprised at all, it was going accordingly as we planned later today. We were at the apartment of my sister-in-law. I had been here a few times as much as I could remember when I used to see everything fine. She has not yet moved in with her family though it was fully well furnished. It was a duplex.

"Wow! Let me not be persuaded by my happy thoughts". I had a Vitrectomy today and I am clueless about my future now more than ever.

My arms were gently held by my wife as she mildly struggled to get me out of the car. I stepped out of the car without ease, my wife guided me through the parking lot.

"Hold on. Lift your foot, we are about to get into the elevator". She said.

I imagined it to be an elevated porch and a single step up, I would be in front of the elevator's door. I felt foolish if the entire floor was moving upwards; it meant I was already inside the elevator and it was ascending to its destination on the fourth floor.

I was once again guided and gently held onto my arms by my sweet wife out of the elevator. All the time she's been very careful about my steps yet I couldn't shake the feeling that something unknown might hit my face or me as I walked every step. Finally, she knocked at the door, she even managed to get my shoes off.

There she stood, and one of my sisters-in-law opened the door. I was sitting on the soft couch, making myself comfortable, and I could hear two sisters chatting about the day.

"How are you feeling now?", my brother-in-law asked.

I simply replied, "I feel nothing only hopeful that everything will work out well".

"It will ", he assumed.

How void I was from inside I couldn't tell anybody. The wicked feeling of helplessness and fear engulfed my thoughts. No matter how hard I struggled to calm my thoughts. I felt tragic from the inside. The question of" Why me?" was haunting me profoundly. At that time, I wasn't sure about the answers because I had not yet met my Massiah who could answer all the questions I had going on in my head.

 Something interesting happened then. I was in the bath with my wife, our bodies colliding under the warm shower and sharing the pure ecstasy of being a man and a woman. Well, before any naughty thoughts hit your mind, let me clarify; I cannot let water get into my recently operated eye. I had to be very cautious about following the post-surgery instructions. So did my wife as well. She guided me to the basin where I could wash my hands and remove the dirt. Further, she undressed me though I couldn't get a real bath, she gently poured water from the mug down my neck standing behind me perfectly like a mother bathing her toddler. It was prescribed that water shouldn't get into the operated eye even after removal of the bandage, which was the following day. I had to stay without pouring water on my face or say technically can't wash my face at least for the first ten to twenty days but in my case, it was advised to follow till one month. Yes, of course, I can wipe my face off any dirt or that tropical greasiness from my face.

Note: The most crucial time is the post-surgery hours. It is essential to follow all the advice prescribed for the healing process to start effectively.

I was guided gently to the bed after that partial shower. I thought my back needed a real bed to lay on. The bed was ready indeed, I could not see but reasonably it should be and my sister-in-law didn't disappoint me as she already prepared the bed perfectly ready to be devoured by me. I assumed the facedown position for the first time, technically a " prone position," and I expected to lie on my back. what a mess! I realized that lying on my back or the usual sleeping position was no longer an option. I had a new, rather not-so-normal position to spend some of the hours of my life. I had to adapt to this new, unconventional way of resting. Life during facedown was inevitable, if there was an alternative, I doubt there wasn't any.

This position helps to ensure that the gas bubble or silicone oil used to hold the retina in place remains in the correct location to aid the healing process. In my case, silicon oil was implanted into my eye.

Life during facedown

After a few seconds on my face downward, I realized that my neck began to ache. In addition, I could feel the effect of anesthesia evaporating, and the slow stink of a needle kind of sensation started to build in my eye.

"I might have pain in my eyeball now," I told my wife.

To my ignorance, I was more concerned about my pain, but I didn't realize that the coming days would be a pain in my ass. Yeah! Maintaining the Prone position was a bonus.

To my words, my wife didn't reply, and I was pretty much sure that she was willing to help me ease the pain, but technically she didn't know what could be done except to put the eyedrops carefully, and I took the few pills that were prescribed in time.

The dinner was served to me at maybe around seven pm, which was too early for the customary of urban lifestyle. But there it was, but I could not find the dinner plate or the delicious food on it. I could only see an array of black and black. As I was experiencing total darkness, a hand started to feed me with that tasty food, and my hunger started to spike harder. I was emotionally driven to think for a while that perhaps it was better if I could eat with my own hands; it would have been a much more fulfilling effect. When it comes to eating rich, I would eat like a 'Gourmand', which in case most of the witnesses would have suggested. I was fond of rich that's why maybe I usually ate most of my time at home only. This time too I was enjoying every bite of it though I was fed like a child. Maybe it took less than half an hour and I was fed with the last bite of the dinner plate. Well, I was not calculating the time but I assumed it instinctively when I was lying in a prone position the first night. My medication was taken care of by my wife, and as I was positioned in Facedown, I could feel that weird squeezy kind of sensation in my eyeball once again. It felt as if my eyeball had taken the shape of a squeezy and bouncy jelly. The Prone position was easy, sit with a facedown, eat with a facedown, sleep with a face down, and walk with a face down, or else what? That's it. I didn't realize that things that seem easy are often hard to do. It may be less than an hour when my neck gave up. The pain in my eye was building strongly. pain has got my proper address and was an uninvited guest tonight. I never thought that I would have to bear so much pain in my operated eye. My neck was showing its tantrums too. There was no one to blame; even if there were, it would have been an easy escape. I kept tossing and turning, shifting from one side of the bed to another. I mean, hilariously I was shifting on all the sides of the bed to get the elusive most needed simple sleep. I called my wife to feed me the painkiller.

"I feel like if my eyeball is on fire "

I had earlier gone through some of the case studies on the internet and even YouTube. I didn't get my hands on any record clarifying post-surgery discomforts, yes, pain would be there but to that discomforting level, I didn't expect it. I knew the surgery would be painless which was obvious for most medical surgeries but expecting one's own body to resist so much assault would be foolishness. It has its ways of saying to stop it now and maybe pain was part of it. That's all I could say to myself.

I prayed for relief, and the painkiller I guessed had started to do its job. Maybe after half an hour, I felt a little relief and fell asleep. Before that, I adjusted two pillows on both sides of my head to stop it from tipping as I fell asleep. I ensured the facedown position with this little " jugar" or say " jury-rigging". I wasn't aware of the available solutions online, nor did my wife know about something called a "facedown pillow". It was something which cold had a great remedy like a "Messiah "in my journey. But that was it, it happened and I maintained a facedown with my two darling pillows every time I had to go for a nap or deep sleep. I would not suggest that any fellow retinal detachment patient adjust during face-down with "rigged" solutions. Still, I would suggest getting proper resources to continue the face-down journey in a comfortable zone. The "prone position" is the most crucial factor in the healing process. If I had to split the healing process into 80/20, 80% would be maintaining a face-down position carefully and consistently as prescribed, and 20% would be the medication, diet, and lifestyle.

Facedown was not easy, man. I had to live with it for more than a month, but it is not obvious that every eye specialist would prescribe it for a long duration, like a month or more than a month. In most cases, it would be for ten to fifteen days, my case was different. And so the whole treatment process varies by the kind of retinal detachment or damage one has. I continued facedown for one month and it was unexplainable how I managed thirty days and nights. The following day I woke up, and the pain in my eye was not completely gone yet, it was there but I felt it was slowly subsiding. My last night's sleep was kind of not so okay, but it was more of a battle. I would say. My sister-in-law served the lovely breakfast while my wife fed me gently. The appointment was at 8;15 am. I was ready and I was hopeful that I would get back my vision as soon as the bandage was removed from my eye just like in the movies. A blind man could start sighting as soon as the operation was done and the bandage was removed, "kaboom!" There it was. I didn't know what the script of a movie could demand. In the present context, I was desperate for light; unlike if both eyes were working well and you needed only one eye to operate, then I couldn't really imagine what I would have expected or what anybody would have expected. But I was desperate to see the things again back in their perfect shapes and sizes, yes, I wanted to see things not that somber darkness. I hoped I would see things once again, but didn't realize that the journey had just begun. We reached the eye institute, and by we mean my brother-in-law and us. He just happened to pick up something that I had forgotten now so he decided to give us a ride on his way. I could hear my wife asking for the wheelchair at the entrance of the huge building. I still remember every detail of that place. I had been visiting regularly for more than a decade. I could imagine the hustle around me, but I just couldn't realize how the eye problems in people had significantly risen. I was guided to the loyal wheelchair once again, and I had to put my trust in the guy who drove me to the post-surgery ward, where the bandage from the eye had to be dressed off.

I can't express how my heart was pounding at that time. The imaginative fear of losing the eyesight forever of the only eye with sight was no less than walking on the tip of a blade. I was hoping miracle the expected one but after the dressing of the eye, I could see all is nothing but blurry, diffused lights. What just happened? I couldn't believe it, I was in tears inside. I prayed to the omnipotent, or rather, I complained about it. I didn't ask for it, but there was no reply. Once again, I had to put back my unanswered questions with myself, and the doctor entered the room. Yes, it was the guy who did the surgery, I could say from hearing the voice. He did what needed to be done and exclaimed, "The surgery was good". I somehow gathered my courage and asked him how long it takes for me to see things again.

"We really can't say, maybe a week or more than a few weeks," he gently replied.

I was not satisfied, but I trusted his words. I could only hope and trust my faith. To be hopeful in hopeless times. I was carried out to the lobby in the same way I was carried to the post-surgery ward. My wife booked a cab on Uber. Very soon we reached back to the apartment since it was morning hour and there was not much rush on the road. Now what? I thought. The answer was simple: continue with the medication and maintain the face down. I had an appointment in five days. My wife gave a call to my mom, giving her the very details of what the doctor told us and how my condition was. I was missing my baby girl.

"She is fine," my wife reported to me.

It was hard to disbelieve the fact of what children mean to parents. They were the epicenter of their hearts; I realized then how I was missing her face and that smile. I was worried if she felt the same way, missing her dad and mom. Life was cruel at its best but I was trying to disbelieve it. I had seen life to be always beautiful and so young. Okay, let us keep that sight for a while and concentrate on facedown yeah! the 'star of the hour'.

Life during facedown won't be easy, I could say from my own experience but lucky you if you had both eyes working well, though not superbly. Still, you could watch your favorite mobile phone, whatever you like, while lying facedown. Well in that case, I was lucky too, cause I didn't have to keep myself amused or entertained while facedown. I or anybody needed to maintain the "Prone position "sincerely as prescribed by the eye surgeon precisely. Let me clarify, "Prone position" plays the most heroic role in putting your operated retina back in its position in most cases, so, facedown shouldn't be taken lightly as fun, but it's part of the healing process. I couldn't suggest what could be done more to ease the discomfort because I didn't think much about it except to do it 24 hours with an occasional break of a minute or two. Going through pain and discomfort was all part of it. Our body slowly adapts to it as we do it more often and it was not something newly discovered fact about the possibilities our body can do. Perhaps a reminder that all will be well. My first few days were exhausting, and I struggled a lot. The peace I wanted was all disrupted, I couldn't sleep properly, couldn't watch anything and walking was nowhere in the scene. I had to rely on my wife even to move from my bed to the washroom. I had spent my days lying facedown mostly on the bed. I tried not to get my thoughts into imaginary sabotage about my predicament, my sad situation, and the unwanted fear.

After a week, I gradually felt not so much, though a little comfortable, while facedown. I didn't have to force a conscious effort to get into the act; it became normal, like the daily activities of any given day. However, lying face-down after a meal caused mild discomfort in breathing. It seemed I was doing good in the "Prone position". I started to like the face-down position ridiculously. It had only been a week, and I knew I still had a long way to go.

I assumed there are a few things to follow and one could do during facedown:

1. Initially, it seems very difficult but tell your conscious mind that you have to do it for the number of days as prescribed and instructed so that the healing of retinal detachment starts correctly.

2. Forget about your amusement or entertainment, it would be damn frustrating but be ready to accept the fact that you had a retinal

detachment, and it's not okay to take the "Prone position" lightly. It had to be done correctly.

3. You would be most lucky if you had someone who could understand your situation, so look for someone to talk with to brighten up your mood instead of watching a mobile phone or even reading a book. You could also listen to the radio or podcasts or music if you like.

4. To ease the discomfort, one could have a facedown pillow and I am sure that there are other retinal detachment patient aids available on the market.

5. Be careful not to trip on your sides while you are asleep. Make sure that somebody watches your position, or else you will be on your own to maintain the best.

6. Avoid walking even in your home. Try to be in one place and maintain the position without letting your head move or turn so don't think of any activity that may involve turning your head even slightly, put your focus on facedown for the best recovery.

7. Be aware that maintaining a facedown position helps the air bubble reposition the detached retina. Therefore, following this recommendation for a few days or even longer is crucial for recovery.

8. Any instance of discomfort in the eye or elsewhere, get back to your eye surgeon for the

best advice. Stay away from people giving expert opinions on retinal detachment even if someone has experienced retinal detachment before, Every case is unique and requires personalized treatment. Be patient.

On the fifth day after the surgery, I went back to the eye institute as I had an appointment. My vision had not improved, not even a slight. I was sitting with my wife in the same old OPD where I got to know about this retinal detachment. We used to talk a lot when we were out together but it was different that time. We hardly exchanged words, and I was listening to the hustle around me. I was in a Facedown position. I could see lights in the blurry form and distorted, someone had never seen before. Barely distinguishable in their hazy form. I was assuming, it would end as soon the Ophthalmologist checked my eye and put some eye drops, I would see clear light again. I was sitting on the stall and the surgeon, Mr. Barman was checking my eye through the Ophthalmoscope.

"Now I would put a few eyedrops and your eye will be as fine as ever", he exclaimed.

That's what I thought. I was expecting something miraculous to happen and all I could see was blurry and foggy light. With a heavy breath, he said, "Okay the retina is all good and I'll review it after a week."

That's it. The expected miracle didn't happen nor did he put eyedrops in my eye. I couldn't argue with anyone for this delay in returning my precious vision. We left the eye institute While sitting on the co-driver seat, I saw everything in its most disfiguration forms. It was more like if I was underwater and trying to figure out what lay underneath. I was too dramatic in my thoughts at that time but that's how it went, I didn't know what to do. After a week or a few more days, I started noticing the change in my vision. The things were not visible clearly but I could make out their colors, like the color painted on the wall of my room, the doorway, table, chairs, so literally whatever was there. It brought relief in those suffocating moments. The first sign of hope I was longing for was happening. At least I was coming to a workable condition, I mean I could see partially enough to go to the washroom and come back, and I could have my meals with my hand now—no longer needed to be fed by my beloved wife Unlike if my other eye would have worked, things would have been much different for me.

I did my third eye check-up after a week and this time things were not as gloomy as it was before. As said before, my eyesight had started to change. I could now see the less hazy light and could make out what I was looking at. Even on returning to the apartment, I did see things around much clearer, though not in good shape, yeah! I could see.

On returning to the place we were staying, my wife and I decided to move to our own home. Most likely, I could walk on my own now and could see the things around me, though not clearly like a normal person would with normal vision. But still, I could manage now.

"let's go back to our home now, I think things will be better off from now on", I said to my wife.

She agreed too without hesitation. I didn't know what came next but I was destined to get back to my own house and to my bed. I was thinking about our baby girl, too. It's been over a week since we left her with her grandmother. During all those days, I struggled to maintain a face-down position but there wasn't a day I didn't speak about our baby girl to my wife. Finally, I would see her now and hold her in my arms. I was excited about this moment of reunion with my baby girl as if I was about to meet her after a decade, which was not. It was only a week, and I was clueless about mentioning it again. I was in fear and that unexplainable thought of what would come next. The answer was simple: I had to stick with the prescribed routine until the next checkup. Which was twenty days after the surgery.

What to expect from the surgery?

In the beginning, I had thought nothing much about the whole process of the healing of the retina that was detached, but was more concerned about getting back to normal life as soon as possible. I wasn't aware that I had real damage to my eyesight. I knew that I had to retain the prone position, be careful not to let the operated eye get infected, and do the medication as prescribed. It was a nightmare situation to stay blind like that.

As of now, the number of my glasses has increased a lot, and if not worse, I cannot see things clearly without putting them on. It has significantly impacted my day-to-day life. The lost portion of my eyesight could have been saved if my retinal detachment had been detected at the earliest.

I had come to that conclusion, but in my later years, while going through some research for this book, I realized that usually, a retinal detachment is an eye condition where the detached retina could be reattached in one single surgical procedure but sometimes multiple procedures may be required. The success of a detached retina depends on the amount of tear the retina has and the amount of scar tissue formed in the retina. If the 'Macula', the central point of the retina were not affected vision would be good. If the Macula were detached for a longer period, some amount of vision would be lost; it would be like 20 /200. which would be legally blind. It would take several months or a couple of years to determine the amount of vision a person may get back. The success of a retinal reattachment surgery depends mostly on the amount of the retinal tear in the eye. The crucial point is the healing period. A lot depends on the healing process and the person's lifestyle as well.

My expectations after the first surgery—yes, you read it right. My first surgery was not a total failure, but it wasn't fully done yet, as I heard from my eye surgeon later. I had three surgeries. I will come to that part, but now for my expectations. nothing unusual I was expecting. I only hoped to return to normal life, which meant getting out of that uncomfortable position and eyesight. I was impatient to get back to business.

We hired a taxi to take us to our home on a hilltop. The road was a real deal. It was a narrow one-way path winding uphill, and as I had mentioned earlier, we were still new to that small, close-knit community of people living there. I wouldn't say I was fond of living on that hilltop, away from the hustle of city life. It was much worse because of the road condition, which worsens on rainy days. We were lucky, I would say, that there wasn't any rainfall in the last few days. As I exited the car, I heard the familiar voices echoing with concern for my well-being. My wife helped me climb the stairs leading to our home.

I sat on the couch and I asked about our baby girl to my mom, "She had just fallen asleep ", she replied.

My wife had bought most of the items that our baby girl loves to devour. It had been a week since we had seen our apple of the eye. We wanted to make her happy and forget about the days of separation by offering her the goodies her mother had brought. I walked into the bedroom, and my baby girl was asleep in the comfort of her bed, unaware of the fact that her mom and dad were back in the home. I watched her for some time, but I couldn't see her innocent face due to my blurred vision. I couldn't change by force or by my wish what was happening with my vision, now I had to carry on the face-down position for the next few more days.

I didn't exchange many words with anybody back home; I had nothing much to say or talk about. Maybe I only replied to my mom, who was concerned about my vision. After a while, I felt the urgency to empty my stomach while doing the "shit", I recalled something I got to know from the internet that I should not strain when defecating. It was not something advised by my doctor, but I could not ignore the fact that it might have some bad impact on the healing of the detached retina. As I was taking a shower, I had to be careful not to let water anyhow get into my operated eye and it was obvious, but I felt like I needed to do the thing any average guy would think who hadn't had sex for more than a week. I hadn't had sex for more than a month, I guess, and this surgery had ruined all the expectations. I knew the waiting would be long.

"O, come on, you have many years left to have sex enough, " my conscious mind told me.

It was that I had to focus more on the smooth healing of my detached retina than anything, since I was surviving with that only working eye. I didn't want to go blind. I came out of the bathroom. Lying face down on my bed in a separate room, I tried to calm down my thoughts for a while and tried to take a nap.

What you should expect from the Surgery?

1. In most normal scenarios, the first surgery would do the work and reattach the detached retina. However, some had to go for multiple surgeries. If so then don't be heartbroken.

2. The type of treatment depends on the degree of retinal detachment and sometimes the surgeon's preference so don't compare your condition with someone else.

3. Be hopeful and follow the routine prescribed to you

4. Don't keep unrealistic expectations; be ready to face whatever comes.

I almost lost all hope when I found out that I had to go for a second surgery. It was as if my fate was destined to ruin whatever years I had left with my life. I was scared what if I had to live a blind life? So do my family. I blamed my parents for such a plight. The next six months after returning to my home were the most difficult, at least for me which I have tried to elaborate on in the following chapter.

Chapter -four

Fighting my Demons

Dr. Jacob Bolotin's journey to pursue a career as a physician was full of grief and extraordinary achievements. Going through a hard process of sleepless nights and dedication to get a degree would sound normal for any medical student, but Jacob Bolotin had to go through much more than his blindness making him unsuitable for work. At first, he faced criticism and denial of the recognition and appreciation he deserved.

He was born to Polish Jewish immigrant parents in Chicago in 1888. His life story was something we could imagine or see only in movies, most likely it was hard to believe unless you had met him in person. He would be the first physically disabled person or say a blind person to join the medical school and would become a licensed physician. He was born at a time when there were no programs dedicated to blind or disabled persons, Perkins Braillers, or any other mediums. yet, he endured and believed in his ability. He was once the best typewriter salesman in a company before he was one of the outstanding well-known heart and lung specialists.

How come a person who was blind by birth could be unimaginably a licensed physician and excellent at what he does.? Normally I could imagine a person blind to be in a position where he would be unsuitable for working and might end up depending on someone throughout the lifespan. I had seen blinds begging and singing in the streets and the railway stations. Sightings of blinds working in normal jobs or medical institutions are rare. Similarly, Dr. Bolotin was an exception too. But he was not the only one achieving a rare accomplishment despite his Blindness, if we look around globally there are many other examples of greatness achieved by people despite physical disabilities and wonders the world with delight but the harsh reality is we all wear our own shoes. Such rare life stories grab our attention and to some point, they motivate us and inspire us to carry on the burden of life without hesitation to go to the extent where we fall apart if life demands and get the courage to rise again. But, the practical reality of every man is different and so do our circumstances.

No matter how I tried to encourage myself for better times, somewhere I could hear a voice giving me a downbeat feeling and fearing me with all the imaginative consequences of something I never wanted. The struggle entirely seemed one-sided but it wasn't over yet.

My wife had fifteen days of leave from her office duties and had to return to her job in the coming week. My mother was too anxious about her husband back in our hometown, it's been more than two weeks since she had come. Occasionally her husband would call and ask about my progress and she would reply with a heavy sigh whatever she had witnessed and understood. I knew somewhere she was praying to her God seeking a blessing or maybe a miracle to happen. At that point in time I was dubious about God's wish and the ignorance of my parents. I had started to develop an indifferent attitude toward God and them for my whatever the condition. I wished that God had much better plans for me and that my parents could have taken much better action for my eye treatment earlier.

Our search for a miracle

I still remember an event regarding one self-acclaimed miracle man who claimed that he had been blessed to cure diseases that modern medicines had not successfully treated. He had that "tree of cure" which has the remedial extract to cure all kinds of diseases. This great news like wildfire reached my hometown too. The place was an hour's drive away. Along with my mother and me, another family joined and we set on our way to meet that miracle man. My mother was hopeful that someone would finally get me back my vision of my right eye. On hearing my mother's expectation I was fool enough to believe whatever that miracle man could do. I had my expectations too. After an hour, our rented car took a left turn from the highway to an unsurfaced road and we were informed that we had to cover another distance of one mile and we would be at that man's doorstep. No one exactly knew where the house of that man was and at that time, Google Maps was not in trend, it was on my 10th standard in 2000. It was only five years since mobile phones were introduced in India and Google Maps services was not launched yet. We had to navigate by asking every passerby and we did find his place after all he had become quite popular.

It was a hut in a rural background with a "Pandal" in the yard. An enormous crowd surrounded the Pandal means it was not large enough to hold all the visitors. We were doubtful of our chances if we could be able to meet him that day. On seeing the crowd, I didn't feel any spiritual vibe; rather, it felt as if we were at a carnival. Indeed, it was no less than a carnival, a carnival of a miracle man.

As we waited there for the blessed man, it had been more than an hour, so I decided to explore the surroundings during the given leisure. Walking among the gathered crowd, I saw the helplessness of the people, families, and whoever was there. They all came with a hope which was not real at all. I was persuaded by it too expecting a miracle from that miracle man only with a hope to see again. We were too innocent to believe in such a Godly thing in the age of modern medicines. Perhaps believing in an unreal belief made us all gather in that unknown rural side with a common purpose.

I couldn't find any breathtaking sites except open fields with cows and buffalos grazing on that sunny day. The wind was mild but cold, and I could see a whirl of dry leaves winding around. The wait was over, my ma called and told me that they were going to stay the night there.

 "They had talked to one of the coworkers and got an appointment in the morning the following day. Coincidentally, a relative of our neighbour was a native of that village and had requested to stay the night at their home".

"It's good, at least we are guests tonight", I replied.

We had country chicken for dinner and some rice beer, a popular beverage. My sleep was quite okay. I shared the room with the elder son, and no sooner did I fall asleep than I didn't remember. The rooster alarmed the sun rising the next morning, we all were heading for that hut after our simple breakfast of black tea and some biscuits.

 "The sight was not so different from yesterday", I said.

It was like the same people waiting for their turn, fixed there waiting for a miracle to happen in their lives, expecting a cure for their agony of carrying the burden of some diseases. We entered the same yesterday's "Pandal", my ma talked to the co-worker, and we were asked to give him a second or a minute. Likewise, after some seconds or minutes, he came back and asked my ma and our neighbour to follow him to the small room next to the "pandal". I was not supposed to follow the adults, so I did wait for my ma to get me the news that my ears wanted to hear. I waited again, but not very long for that time, I saw my ma and our neighbor walking out of that room. I inquired what he said.

"The man was very polite and humble. It was mindful talking to him", she replied.

"Okay, it's fine, ma, but what did he say about my eye? Could he restore my lost eyesight?" I exclaimed.

"He had that kind of a holy tree planted in the middle of a single-room hut, the rumor was that it came out on its own and had been giving out some sort of fluid or sap that has medicinal or unexplainable significance that can cure most of the diseases. The man said he had a vision and was visited by the Goddess in his dream who instructed him to follow what she says next. So, he was doing whatever had been told to him by the Goddess. He could cure the diseases of body pain, headache, kidney stones, and many more, but cannot get back the vision of a blind eye. Basically, what he meant was that nerve-related sickness he cannot cure so there was no by any chance, he could take care of my eye." That's what he had to say when my mother told him about our visit.

So, our expedition in search of that miracle ended in dismay. Not for our neighbor, who had found the solution for his ill son. He would bring his son to that man for the next week.

From then on, my parents never talked about miracles from any miracle men. I never realized or didn't understand how heavy it would have been on their hearts not to be able to reverse what had caused such a predicament. But it was more painful to be in that situation, which I never realized or cared about until now.

Understanding the patient's mental state

"Life will get you down if you don't look up."

The days back at home were not easy at all. I assumed that I had gone through too much as a person with retinal detachment and the pressure of parental as well as a family man's obligations.

My wife returned to her office duties, and my mom returned to her hometown. It was only a few days, more than a month after the first surgery. From now on, I had to take care of the household and our baby girl. We couldn't rely on anybody else, and we couldn't afford a housemaid or expect a relative or a distant cousin to come and stay with us for some days. Life was busy, so it was for everyone.

The normal routine life started and I had to struggle which was obvious for my eyesight. Every morning my wife would do her part to prepare the day's meal and do the other cleaning and washing. After she left for her office, it was me and our baby girl all on our own back at home. The initial days were good but slowly the boredom of doing the repeated things started to consume me and my wife and there were indifferent arguments that started to build up like between any normal couple. I couldn't get out of the blame game situation and it was slowly turning me into somebody melancholic from the inside. It was something that I had created for my own, I had that indifferent attitude towards my parents, my wife, my fate, and almost everything in my life and it had impacted my temper to a great extent. I felt like everyone else life was sorted but not mine. I had only suffered. I was moody and had mood swings most of the time. It was like almost a spoiled child would do for the sake of anything that the child demanded from his parents. My wife had to bear it mostly so did our baby girl. "Well! hold on", I never physically lost my temper or did something unexpected that could have harmed my wife and anybody near me yes I did break a few negligible items back at home at that time.

Every day was a new struggle for me, that's what I felt. Handling household duties like preparing a meal for our baby girl and me, occasionally sweeping and mopping the floor, and doing the dishes were in the routine. This was not something I had ever done before but this time I felt it was too heavy for me with that blurred vision and a dubious feeling. The uncertainty and fear if it didn't work. My occasional mood swings had something to do with the retinal detachment and it was not something any Psychiatrist or a counsellor notified me about it. If I see now and then, I can't disbelieve the fact that healing depends not only on the person's mindset and a strong will but also few motivational words from those who are close by. Words can do a lot during the recovery period but sadly I didn't feel it in my wife's presence or even anyone else. I was consumed too much with this unwanted predicament of my own. It was undoubtedly my stupidity when it had always been that most likely my problems would get noticed but would never be felt by someone else the way I felt or imagined about it. It was totally normal that way, that's how people work, in fact, the world works.

My perception of the negative side was heavier than the positive aspects which I hardly noticed. I was not ready to accept the fact that my life wouldn't be the same as it was before and it had saddened me a lot. At times I got so sad that tears started to roll down my cheeks and I couldn't help but blame God and my fate. So my days back at home didn't have a good start, it seems like that from my perspective but I must tell you that I hardly understood that "Problems are inevitable", its like never-ending. You cannot drag somebody to be on your side all the time when it is entirely your fight alone. I cannot change what has to happen. Life has its ways of doing what it does.

My mother stayed with me for a few days and she regularly took care of my medication. My wife did a fantastic job by printing out the day's schedule of all the different medicines and eyedrops with the time slot, and made it hang just above the bed where I slept. It helped my mother in her late fifties to easily recall the medication schedule that I was prescribed. It was always a great comfort to have family around during any medical or health challenges. Well, it was all good, but only what they missed out on unknowingly was that I needed mental support as well. I needed to flush out my thoughts and share them with someone who could listen. Even I wanted to share it with my beloved wife but I hesitated because she had a busy schedule, was managing most and had her belief system which I didn't want to intrude on moreover she was in grief too I believe but now I realize it was an unfair act that I didn't tell her what was going on in my head and my thoughts.

There was a study conducted to investigate "Mood disorders" or "Mood swings" of people who experienced retinal detachment by using the "National Health Insurance Database", in Taiwan. The study included participants who had been diagnosed with Retinal detachment and were the main study whereas another group without any history of retinal detachment.

The outcomes related to mood disorders after a retinal detachment included in the study were:

1.   Psychiatric outpatient departments

2.   Behavioural therapy

3.   Sleep or anxiety-related disorders

4.   Major depressive disorders

A total of 4,129 participants with a Retinal Detachment and 16,516 with no Retinal Detachment were enrolled in the study. It was found that patients with a recurrent RD who received more than two treatments and female patients with RD who needed surgery showed a higher probability of mood swing disorders in comparison to Non-Retinal Detachment participants. So the study concluded that those with Retinal Detachment who needed surgical intervention were at higher risk of developing mood disorders (reference: my.clevelandclinic.org/health/treatments/2440 2-vitrectomy)

The reality was that I did not have any intense mood disorders as I had ignorantly assumed; however, it was more of a pessimistic approach towards life and my own stupidity. It was the moment when I thought all my dreams and hopes were shuttered and stripped away from me. This shadow of gloomy nature stayed with me until I got my new power lenses.

After a month at home, I was done with my face-down position, and in the recent checkup, I was assured that my retina was settling to its normal position. It was a relief but I didn't see much change in my sight, it had that blurry effect and it stayed for the next month as well in addition, straight lines seemed not straight, a wavy kind of pattern I could see whenever I gazed at the window panels, door panels or even the simple objects like a stick in my hands or the ceiling fan. It seemed as if all these had a band or wavy shapes. I didn't understand anything at all at that time; moreover, I could feel my sight was weird. At night, when I go to bed and turn off the light, I can see a kind of flickering light for some seconds and even a shadow like something which I cannot explain when I move my pupils, though these stay for some seconds, but such occurrences made me fabled and fearful. I could only imagine myself in a helpless situation without any hope or answers. I couldn't recall what made me try not to accept the way it was. My life was pretty average and I had some complaints until this retina thing happened and shattered all my dreams and plans for the future.

"Things have unexpected ways to start"

I wanted to start something in the online space. I had some plans and hopeful expectations. Some ideas to make my life meaningful and a regular income stream. I taught at a school before putting off that job to take care of our baby girl and the other household activities. At that time, I didn't feel much about changing jobs and never dreamt that my life would be regretful like this, regretting not starting what I wanted to do. The boom in the online space after the COVID-19 pandemic inspired me to find a place in the online space, as I was getting started to take care of the household full-time, I never expected something unexpected would happen. I was supposed to feel relaxed and calm my thoughts, but the ambitious me inside always had a reason to break loose. Moreover, the result of going through three consecutive eye surgeries damaged my thoughts pretty badly.

After three months, I got to know that I had to go for another eye surgery, almost in the same process where the silicon oil would be implanted again, and after one month, if everything went well, it would be removed.

"No way! Another surgery", I thought, but it had to, so once again I tested the surgery table and the pain after surgery night. The weird vision for the next few days or more, and yep! The old facedown position. However, the second time was prescribed only for fifteen days. I actually felt good about it this time, keeping myself in a "Prom position" not for as long as it was previously. It was only that I felt comfortable thinking that obviously, things would be better from now on. I had gone through too much, so faith had to be on my side now or else I could do nothing but be more pathetic than ever.

In the later days, I realized that a positive mindset is required to be able to overcome all the imaginative stuff that I had infused myself with. I had to trust the process and the treatment. Just imagine if I had had a retinal detachment ten or twenty years back, it could have been a different, worse scenario. I required something to believe in, and that only idea had smoothed up the situation in many ways. If it had happened like that, then I guess it would have had a much better perspective for my vision, but I could have worse situation due to slow technological upgradation in the medical sector in my country. The earlier a retinal detachment is diagnosed, the better the chances are of getting fewer complications in gaining vision or retaining the same amount of eye vision. I couldn't stop myself from thinking of myself in an alternative universe where I was living a life that I thought of losing here.

Faith in the almighty

"When all doors are closed, there still remains one door opened for all, that's the door to God."

One night not disbelieve that I am not a spiritual or a religious individual. I had a few occasional instances when I hardly ever visited temples in my city, but I cannot deny the presence of someone omnipotent and omnipresent. I don't visit temples or actively participate in all the poojas regularly, yet I have never disbelieved his omnipresence. My mother, on the other hand, was a loyal devotee of Lord Shiva. I had never known her that she would miss a day without having a bath in the morning and lighting up the earth lamp at our home's "tampon", a wooden structure where all the idols of deities are kept together. It's a common thing in every household in India. I had grown up seeing her do that, and somehow this old habit of hers had reflected in me too. I proudly can say I do have a "Thapona" at my home too, and sometimes I miss offering my prayers and lighting up the earth lamp.

The day when my first surgery was on, my mother faithfully trusted the ways of God, and like a loyal devotee, she promised that she would visit one of the spiritual sites of lord Krishna, namely "Vasudeva thaan" in the upper Brahmaputra valley, for a thankful gesture if the lord listens to her prayers. I never doubted God's will, and if the prayer of my mother had ever been heard. The news was that my first surgery was a success in terms of putting the detached retina back in its place and after three months, my eyesight has not improved yet. I had developed seeing things in double (diplopia) and even in some instances, it appeared triple, particularly when I looked a normal room light bulbs or a burning candle. I thought that it would get better when I would get my glasses with the new corrected power. The reality was different, I was suggested another "Vitrectomy" (when I heard it from the surgeon, I smiled sarcastically in my mind and complained to God). My family and I had to swallow our expectations once again and be nothing but hopeful and set the prayers on.

The realization of a change

Something unexpected happened to me as well, apart from the second surgery; this time, I was miraculously not worrying too much or feeling the agony of my circumstances. Maybe it was more because I didn't have to brainstorm for arranging the expenditures or worry about the medical bills, which, on the other hand, my dear wife was making sure that there wouldn't be any delay in the surgery because of financial misfortune.

There is not a single soul on this planet who has not faced adversity or lived a life without problems. Retinal detachment is not a life-threatening situation. I was making my thoughts too dramatic to be aligned with reality. Yes, I do have only one working eye, and that was affected too. It was nothing new, I was already living with high myopia and glaucoma. Most of the time, I was feeling pity for myself, and it was not sane.

I was determined to keep my thought intake this time and not worry about the uncertainties of life. The second Vitrectomy was done gracefully, I hoped.   As I was led out of the surgery department, the male nurse who was assisting me talked about my long-grown hair. I hadn't had a haircut since my first surgery, and I replied with that old bombastic statement, "We should try on new things in our lives". The truth was, I wasn't trying anything new; rather, I couldn't get a haircut due to the surgery.

Once again, we had to spend the post-surgery night at my sister-in-law's apartment. The night was uncomfortable due to the pain in my eye, yet I survived the night with the hope that there would be a new morning. The following day, I had the check-up after the dressing of the bandage, yep! My eyesight was blurred once again. Being a one-eyed person, it made a big difference in my ability to walk and even do the normal daily things but I survived, and maybe after a week slowly my eyesight got restored, and at that time I could see the things not in double casting any more as it was after the first Vitrectomy but, yet the second surgery has not yet resolved my eyesight. I would see things in that same blurry manner for the next few more weeks, and I thought that it might stay that way forever. One morning, I tried to see my phone for the first time, and I could read the clock time and date on the phone display, and it gave a piece of good news for me and my wife. But the problem was that I had to squeeze my eye a little bit, and if I tried to see with wide-open eyes, it would blur my vision. Next month gone pretty much in the same manner, doing the same old stuff, trying not to be carried away with negative thoughts, and accepting the new change without keeping unrealistic hope for some miracle. I was listening to podcasts and music, motivational videos, and trying to find reasons to laugh and keep the flow of my happy hormones.

I had depressed moments and sad times but these were normal things that could be expected; nobody wants to be sick or bedridden and most likely not be able to see things. Whenever I felt anxious or sad about my circumstances, I would listen to a particular podcast on "Spotify "and most likely you know about it or perhaps read it-"The subtle art of Not Giving a fuck" notably written by Mark Manson. I cannot deny the fact that the book had tremendously impacted my thought process; it had helped me to understand and evaluate the worst scenario that I could think of. My entire focus was focused more on my eyesight only, and why not? who wants to be blind in the middle of his life? I struggled to keep my emotional intake, particularly during the first three months. Unlike other minor eye conditions, it was obvious that a "Retinal Detachment"-Vitrectomy surgery might not give instant results in a short period. Here I can say, "Being patient is the key". Everything else that we expect or hope might not align because retinal detachment is complex, particularly like mine, in the macular end. My eye surgeon did a superb job and I trusted him, so that's what one can do: put one's faith and trust in the process.

 I can't imagine how it felt for someone to maintain life with retinal detachment surgery in terms of balancing office work or business and strengthening the fabric of what keeps life going. I assumed that the complexity around retinal detachment may vary, as do life's circumstances. What I had gone through will not be the same in someone else's case, but we may align with one objective: to see things the way did before. I was always in the blink of losing my entire eyesight, that's what I thought, and this single thought had reasonably overshadowed my positive mindset. The truth is, no matter what we could imagine, the outcome will not be worse than we usually assumed. We will always have that unexpected amount of intolerance towards life's cruelty.

What should be done?

A person who is sick will never feel good about it, and he or she might expect near ones or dear ones to pay attention to them. Emotional support would be expected, and it is favorable for overall well-being and successful recovery. He or she might expect sympathetic attention towards them. You never know how it feels to be bedridden for a sickness unless you have had one. Even a simple cold fever dares to make you feel sick about it as if you would never come out of it for life. In addition, boredom in life tries to make a strong hold on us unless we do something about it. It is difficult for a patient with a detached retina not to think about a hopeful future; believing in a hopeful future is something that keeps us going most of the time. A poor man believes in his hope for a better living, a fisherman hopes for a day of better catch, a soldier hopes for the end of the war, and even Elon Musk believes in the hope for a future with space-science experiments under his lab. Hope is not something that will make a blind man see, but it will keep him going, and accept the harsh life's truth that it is not going to be comfortable, but he will make it to the end line.

Your takeaways-

1.   Don't let the influences of someone who hasn't gone through retinal detachment surgery of any kind persuade your thoughts to lose their ground. No one is going to understand what you have been going through from inside so be grounded.

2.   Self-control seems like an illusion but it's the call of the hour. Calm the emotional flow and focus on something that can help like, listening to music or a valuable podcast or even letting somebody read you out loud any books you prefer to (keeping your eyes away from any stressful activity since reading is an instance eye stressing activity) or else just being yourself and sitting in silence do work.

3.   Meditation can be beneficial. Many of us have heard about its superpower in calming our emotions. Practicing meditation during recovery days would be helpful.

4.   Don't hesitate to speak openly yourself out. People would most likely listen to you.

5.   Start building a positive mindset right from the first day onward when you are diagnosed with retinal detachment. It sounds arbitrary and even crazy, but the truth is most of the healing would be favorable with the right mindset. Healing is not only physical but mental as well.

6.   Under the circumstances of life, there are things that you can't control, so be patient and try not to be upset about it.

7.   Keep your expectations real and don't expect a major change in a short period. (regarding eyesight and life after the surgery)

8.   The routine monitoring periodically after a retinal detachment surgery will be a new addition to life, so embrace it without question. Prescribed routine check-ups have to be followed, which shouldn't make you feel like you are a helpless, sick person. If you don't follow, then you might become a very sick person.

9.   Be happy with the small improvements in your eyesight and rejoice in it with yourself and your dear ones.

10.   I could never say how I would have managed if I had a regular 9 to 5 job and the entire family's expenses depended on me. I am a one-eyesight person so most likely you can better manage the things around you. I wouldn't say to be grateful for whatever eye condition you have but be brave enough to face whatever circumstances follow next for your overall well-being and recovery.

What you can do for the patient

1.   Be helpful and keep your worries aside. Focus on the need of the hour.

2.   Generate a truly positive mindset because your positive mindset will exchange the energy of positivity with the patient as well.

3.   Listen to the patient and encourage the patient to express their fears. if possible monitor the patient's temper and don't get upset because of the circumstance you are in, it is even harder for the patient to cope with the unexpected circumstance no matter how it appears on the surface.

4.   Don't take advice from someone who hasn't the slightest idea about retinal detachment. The best consultation will always come from the medical team.

5.   It is better to light up the mood of the patient and provide emotional support. Try avoiding situations where your thoughts might not align with what the patient thinks. Don't get into a cold war. The patient might be irritating at times.

6.   Take care of the medication and hygiene. Keep the patient in a soothing environment in the

home or wherever and make adjustments whenever needed.

7.   Be available to provide reassurance about their recovery process and the potential outcomes.

8.   Encourage the patient to rely on the support team like family, and friends without shyness or discomfort whenever needed.

9.   Never fail to concern the medical team on any slightest nonrelated abnormal change in the eyesight or other health issues that might arise and need medical intervention.

10.   Provide the patient with clear and accurate information about the eye condition and the potential outcomes.

"Being patient is the key" is not an ordinary, common household saying that you might have heard or ever heard of. Imagine that you were restless and acting mad at anything, most likely when you were trying out something important from your point of view, and your dad called you" Be patient, my boy". At that point at the moment, you might not care about its meaning, but to get the expected end result of what you had been up to. Later, somewhere in your life, in the face of a life situation then you realize the true meaning of being patient. Patience holds the key to accepting setbacks and creating a subtle way for a productive decision.

I had always been a hurry-to-go guy, and I had never tested patience so closely until I got this retinal thing. I thought things would happen at their natural pace, and indeed, they do happen. However, this never meant that they would happen whenever I expected it or wanted them to.

Recovering from a Vitrectomy and witnessing the first sign of improvement usually takes time. It would never be like smashing into a ready meal. It sounds stupid to compare it to eating a ready meal, perhaps that's not silly if I may say that even preparing a meal takes time before it is served on the table. I can't control it, as I'm looking for a better and simpler way to write to highlight the importance of keeping a steady and calm outlook while recovering. Hilariously, we often lose patience, and it is totally normal to not live in the present but dive into the imaginary realm in the future which no one had believed if they did exist. It's normal in the sense that you are hoping for something beautiful for yourself, contrary to all the negative thoughts that might bother you. I did have to go through a lot of negative vibrations in the first initial days, even for months, but all I wanted was a better tomorrow for a poor guy like me. Well, pardon me for exaggerating myself to be a loner with such a pathetic circumstance on the earth, I don't remember how many times I had tried to express my unexpected circumstance and explain the drama that went by for few couple of months but certainly I started taking control of what suits for my better recovery and waited with patience for the outcome.

After going through two surgeries and the final third surgery, I could finally see the picture with certainty that all would be going well from now on. It nearly took one year before I finally got my corrected eyeglasses by the end of 2022. The journey was merely nine months, but it felt like I was getting into an endless tunnel and never coming out of it. I realized that the more anxious I was, I could feel the weight of this burden but honestly, there was nothing I could do and at times there were many things actually I could do and indeed I survived the long wait. Now when I look back, I can see that it was not as long as I had assumed, and wished that I could have understood it at the very start that I needed to be patient and put my faith in the positive aspects. Retinal detachment couldn't be replaced with an anticipated expectation or say a miracle, but with proper diagnosis and suitable treatment that suits the pre-condition of the eye. It's a complicated eye problem that needs complex sets of surgeries, though advanced medical science makes it accessible and quite possible to treat it. The actual results may vary, and one needs to be patient with the whole process for overall recovery. I anticipated the removal of the implanted silicone oil under the Vitrectomy procedure wouldn't take more than three months at the maximum, and then I would be back to my normal routine life; however, it took more than what I had anticipated. It is normal; silicon oil is inserted for retinal detachment repairing surgeries and it would be it for three to six months if any other related complications don't show up so, it indeed demands patience, which I hardly ever thought about until I went for the second surgery. Perhaps at that moment, I could do nothing but trust the process and wait. Recovering from Retinal detachment surgeries takes time, though one may restart life after a few weeks, though with certain limitations. I tried to pinpoint the related reasons and circumstances that might not favor a fast re-entry to routine life after a retinal detachment in the following chapter.

Chapter-Five

Embracing the new horizon of hope

One evening, I was supposed to pick up the milk packets from a local vendor downhill from my place. It had been more than three months since my first eye surgery. Usually, my wife would pick up the milk packets and buy other required items on the way when she returned from her workplace, But that day was the weekend so she didn't have her office open which is quite normal so by evening I decided to pick it up by my own. It had been months since I had left my residence, except during eye checkup calls. My vision had improved too yet I didn't get the corrected glasses. I used to put on a weird-looking pair of black goggles prescribed and given by the eye hospital all the time except at bedtime, I put it down. At one time, it got broken, so my wife got me a pair of better-looking black shades from an eyewear outlet in the city. It was evening time and I was thinking man where on earth was I supposed to put on these black Googles in addition, I was a bit worried too, whether I could walk evenly in the dim light of the sinking sun. There was no street light provision in my locality so I carried a small pocket torch and walked out of my residence. The sky was kissed by the last ray of sunlight for the day, and as it was getting dark, I could see most of the houses lit up with light bulbs. I could see those tiny light bulbs, something like in distorted shapes, but it was much better than how my eyesight was after my first Vitrectomy. As I moved my eye to where I was walking, surprisingly, I could see better even without the corrected glasses. This gave me an unexplainable feeling of joy that I had imagined for a long time.

"Yeah! that's it, it seems I will be fine from here on", I exclaimed in an internal monologue. (I didn't know or was aware of the upcoming second surgery)

Ridiculously, I carried a smile unnoticeable to anybody, and that moment gave me the confidence to be clear of more self-doubts than I had imagined, though not entirely, and I hoped that finally, things would be in place now.

I walked downhill and reached the shop from where I had to pick up the Packets of Milk. I confidently, with my black shades on, asked for it, the man in his white scattered beard, took it out from the refrigerator and handed it to me, he was the owner of that corner shop. Pretty much, we would buy a few of the daily necessities from that shop only, and the owner knew about my eye surgery and asked if I was fine now.

 "I am fine now, but I have to go for another final surgery" (I was expecting the removal of silicon oil)

We talked for a while, mostly about my next medical procedure, and I bought a pack of Lays before saying good night. On my return, I could feel the bouncing of my heartbeat and felt as if I was running out of air; it had been days since I walked like that on a way going uphill. Earlier I depended much on my two-wheeler while commuting, and now it didn't make me happy at all that I had to walk. My wife earlier had warned me about it and exclaimed that no sooner I would start to curse the place in my internal monologue, which I assumed was kind of customary for me whenever I would walk long distances. My bitter thoughts started to come back. It was not that I didn't do physical activities; I used to work out in gyms, ironically, a few years back; however, I was not ready to accept what was happening in my life. Maybe I wanted a reason to blame my body, somebody, or something for no reason.

Most likely, we often don't fit in ourselves in unexpected circumstances that are not in our control, so recovering from an instance surgery is not as simple a deal as it is understood. I had already tried to highlight it in the previous chapter so I don't want to drag you into it once again but What I want you to consider is that going under two consecutive eye operations is not a friendly situation that you would like to encounter as a fellow patient and don't want o see your dear ones go through it as a family or a support person for the patient. I would like to congratulate you if you have endured it; however, in my case, I never truly felt an urgency to understand the fact that the outcome will not fully satisfy me, and feel free enough to acknowledge that my eyesight would not remain the same. I had a few moments that got me feeling a sort of happiness that I didn't have the correct words to express, though it had stayed for a short time.

Raju was a hardworking local Plumber and was happy not for what he did for a living, but he felt happy whenever he was paid for the small or big repair jobs he could find locally. He had hoped to start his service agency and find big plumbing contracts in the real estate. He had ups and downs in his life, but was keeping a straight head.

One day, it was a normal working day. He was at a working site. Nothing was suspicious about that day; he had all his working gear and put all his knowledge into getting the work done until he came across a wall where he had to punch a few holes to connect the concealed pipelines. He started the drilling machine and started punching holes in the marked spot; however, the drilling heads would slip on the tiles mounted wall surface, and he somehow managed it. It was a part of his job, no big deal about it. He managed the first time, the second time, and even the fourth time. On drilling the last hole, he dropped a screwdriver on the floor, and without noticing it, he stepped on it. By the time he realized it, he had an amputated thumb on his right hand. He was rushed to the emergency room nearby.

After a long period of rest for three months, he was back at what he was supposed to do, plumbing but this time he had to compromise on a few things like relying on an assistant for heavy-duty wall drilling or cutting jobs or a few which I might not be able to mention as I don't know much about or anything about plumbing jobs but only assumed that he had to endure pain not only physically but mentally as well. He had a long way to go with this before he could realize his hope of establishing a service agency. I happened to meet him once when our home needed a plumber to fix an issue with the pipeline to the geyser. I was known to him because he was the guy who did the plumbing work on our home, so I could not think of anybody else but him for the job. I couldn't imagine that this guy, who was healthy and doing his job when our house construction was on, would face such a life circumstance. I imagined this guy was no different from me, we both had endured pain and lost, or say fear of losing something we both dearly hold onto, "realizing our dreams".

I don't know much about how he has been doing lately since I met him last; however, my eyesight has not improved on a big scale since it has been more than two years as of now, as I am writing this book. The way my eyesight has developed or improved was not the same as I expected and once felt happy about it, yeah!, it is in workable condition though I can't read books without a reading aid, cannot read the levels on any products or price tags, sign boards or cannot recognize a person by the face unless that person is like two or three feet near me (I mean I cannot make the facial details even with my corrected glasses). This new change felt too heavy in the initial days, but I have adjusted, and my body and mind have adjusted too with the new change. I don't complain about the circumstances anymore; rather, I try to live my life keeping my eye on the safety zone. I could do anything normal, most likely any normal person would do. I read books, watch movies, go to the gym, cook at home, and even ride my two-wheeler; however, the only difference I find is that of poor vision for distant objects, and I could see things in blur without my glasses on. My eyesight was poor before since I had high myopia, well after the latest retinal detachment, nothing changed much except a few more newly prescribed eye drops, and I retired from one activity that is driving a car under any circumstances.

"Whatever amount of eyesight I am left is better than not going fully blind",- that's what I used to say to myself. It took almost one year for me to fully start doing things in a normal way, by which I mean it took almost the mentioned amount of period for me to adjust to the new change in my only working eyesight. Sometimes I would feel a mild kind of headache and would see things in a mild wavy pattern in the beginning, it all occurred like that for high-power lenses which I was prescribed for the corrective glasses.

My final surgery was done just after one month after the second surgery. I didn't have to wait for the scheduled next check-up due to an emergency.

It was that afternoon, after having my meal and feeding my baby daughter, I did the washing dishes part and cleaning up the usual mash-up that I create whenever I enter the kitchen, that's what my wife nags me mostly for, I was trying to get a warm afternoon nap well it was not going as I had planned. I started to feel pain in my operated eye. I felt the kind of mild tension in my operated eye since morning, and I was ignoring it, considering it to be normal, because I have glaucoma, and usually, my eye remains mildly hypertensive most of the time.

However, by the evening, the pain became unbearable. I started to feel nauseous. I was hoping it would subside but nothing happened that way. I wondered if this surgery might have gone wrong; maybe my retina was not reattached well this time, too. I informed my wife about it and told her that I needed to go to the doctor right away. It was almost 4:30 pm, and the doctors' working hours, except in the emergency ward, were about to end. There was no point in expecting my eye surgeon at that hour, so I booked an appointment at the emergency facility. I was with my baby daughter at home, and the working hours of my wife were not done yet. As I was getting myself ready and my baby daughter too, I heard a knock at the front door. It was one of the residents who had heard about my off-colour situation, so most likely my wife informed him about it by a call. I was thankful that he wasn't busy with some other work at the moment so he got ready to drop us both with his motorcycle on the main road from where I booked an Uber to my wife's office. I left my baby daughter with her mom and left for the eye institute (Sri Shankeradeva Nethralaya).On reaching there, it didn't take me more than a few minutes to get in touch with the doctors in the Emergency ward. I was informed about a spike in eye pressure while they checked my operated eye. The check-up lasted for half an hour, going through a few procedures, and finalized an appointment with my surgeon the following day. I was prescribed a few pills to be taken after meals.

I came out and took an Uber once again and was heading to my wife's office. Very soon, we were all in the same cab and headed back to our home. I was sitting in the front row with the cab driver sitting next to me. I was not been able to control my nausea and was feeling as if I was about to throw out anytime soon. Indeed, I puked, I somehow told the cab driver to pull the car aside, and in no time, I opened the door, and that's it. I throw it out by the side of the main road. I was thankful that I could hold it for so long, saving the cab driver from having trouble in cleaning up the mess I created on the dashboard. Yeah! After a few seconds or minutes, I was done and grabbed a bottle of water from my wife. She was worried, which was obvious in the following circumstance. That night, I was anxious once again but decided not to lose my sleep. After all, I had gone through deep moments of despair before, and in reality, I had not seen worse than I had imagined, and a few more rounds would not break me either. I swallowed my daunting thoughts for a better tomorrow. As I lay on my bed to sleep, I remembered God like a hardcore devotee for a better prospect for me the next day.

A day after, I was done with my final surgery and hopefully, the last surgery, and the silicon oil was extracted. During this time, my younger brother accompanied me. He did all the required paperwork and waited till my surgery was done. I was fully blind once again. Next, I was in that same old wheelchair being assisted out of the surgery room. After an hour or so, I was sitting in the front seat of the cab that my brother had booked and we went to his homestay. At that time my brother had a homestay business going. I stayed there for the next five days since I had follow-up check-ups.

Next, whatever followed, I don't want to draw your attention since it was the same damn things happening, which I dramatically tried to elaborate on in the previous chapters in minute details as much as possible. I had spent my initial days in blindness once again, and slowly, maybe after a week or two, I was able to see again. My sight was not exponentially improved, but it was okay, kind of. No matter what job you do or what hobbies you like to spend your time with, vision plays an exceptional role. That part has always been missed from my side. In my earlier days, when I was in high school, I couldn't drive at night hours so my friends had to drive me back home with whatever plans we had at night. It was so funny that at that time, I didn't think it was too serious a thing to be concerned about. I was lucky that I had friends who understood my situation.

In all the chaos of surviving a life, my vision was limited, but it has gone bad after this retinal detachment thing. I don't want to lie about it, but I got a power prescription for the corrective glasses in big numbers, which even only a few lens specialist brands manufacture, like" Nikon". It got heavy in my pocket as well, but it couldn't be compromised.

What to expect after Vitrectomy?

In most cases, a Vitrectomy is as successful as any cataract surgery, though both are done for completely different eye conditions. I said so because retinal detachment is a highly treatable condition, and if it is diagnosed early, vision can be preserved at its best. In my case, I got late, so a good amount of vision couldn't be restored. The sooner it is treated, the better it is.

One must differentiate between expectations and imagination to understand the result of something like Vitrectomy. If you assume that all will be better, then you are not wrong; an early treatment for retinal detachment will not disappoint. However, a late treatment does have consequences. Retinal detachment is a treatable but serious eye condition that has to undergo surgery once or twice, and even in some cases more so, keeping a realistic and practical approach to it, and it would be most beneficial mentally and physically as well. Now, by realistic, I mean you have to understand that you will be most lucky if your vision remains intact as it was before, and if you have to lose some of it, then be grateful that you are not blind. The healing of a detached retina is a purely natural process, with surgery assuring that this process of healing is aided by medical science. Few drugs are meant to treat specific diseases, and they work accordingly;

however, with a detached retina, medicine doesn't do miracles. However, medicine does cure retinal detachments, but surgery is the most effective intervention and the quickest way to treat a detached retina. Under such circumstances and understanding, the result might vary as the degree of retinal detachment. Comparing your expectations to an image of someone else might not be helpful and sound justifiable at all. I do come across people who had detached retinas, and they were treated with Vitrectomy too, but they have better eye vision and better results than mine. Such outcomes have not disillusioned me with something to be regretful of or cry for the rest of my life. I have to be honest that under my eye condition, I couldn't afford to lose vision of my eye since I have only one good eye left. Whatever I would do, I have to be fully dependent on that one eye only.

The most essential thing one could expect is to be able to manage the situations that a detached retina might demand. A proper treatment under an experienced and well-equipped medical facility. To be able to make it to the follow-ups regularly without failing and properly do the facedown without movement. One must understand that surgery doesn't mean it's done with a detached retina; other factors like vision, medication, and proper eye care will play a vital role in assured healing. I can surely understand that the most important concern would be the vision of the eye. The vision in the eye after a

Vitrectomy may vary. Usually, even after three or four months from a successful surgery, it might take more time to fully decide on the amount of vision that would be restored. It has been almost two years since I noticed the exact changes in my eye vision, and currently, I am fully aware of how my vision reacts to things and light. Keeping a straight expectation of getting back into the race track immediately might not sound real; one has to be very patient and act consciously, keeping all the factors in concern. I wasn't fully aware of it and the amount of time it demands, so it had affected my mental well-being for a certain amount of time. The result of a retinal detachment surgery might not be visible in demand or on your expectations, but what has to be done has to be done. A positive mindset, a hopeful attitude, and a calm approach toward the new change would be best.

Your takeaways-

1.   Surgery for a detached retina is as successful as any other general eye surgery but early intervention has to be considered as one most important factors.

2.   Be realistic, early treatment will give better results.

3.   Draw the line between a realistic approach and overly optimistic assumptions.

4.   Healing of retinal detachment depends on a natural process supported by medical interventions.

5.   Comparing personal outcomes with other's experiences is not fair.

6.   Vision restoration may not be always fulfilling but be grateful for the retained vision.

7.   Adaptation is the key, especially for those who already have other severe eye conditions.

8.   Maintaining a positive mindset, and resilience attitude is essential for adapting to any change in vision.

9.   It may take years to fully understand and adapt to the changes in vision after surgery.

10.   A proactive and long-term visionary approach is needed for a positive record

Managing Life

After a Vitrectomy, you might have to wait for two to four weeks before you get back to your work or school and other things that you most likely do. However, there are chances that you might wait for a few more days, weeks, or even months before you become aware of the improvement in vision. You might have to restrict yourself from doing certain things that usually demand more effort from the eyes.

If a gas bubble or silicon oil is implanted in the eye, then certainly your vision will recover at a very slow pace, which might be frustrating sometimes. You would be restricted from taking any air journey and doing heavy-duty work, and even weight-lifting workouts in the gym. Your life will take a brief pause for a while.

All that is mentioned above would be most likely informed to you by your eye care provider, but what you might not be told is how you are supposed to manage your life not only after the surgery but in the long term. What if your vision changes to a great extent after the successful retinal detachment surgery? Well, I am not trying to sound like an expert in this here, but what I am trying to say is that my life's course has changed a lot, which I had already tried to put in words in the earlier chapters. I know what it means when a good amount of vision goes, and the difficulties of life become a bit more difficult. When simple tasks like reading a book or scrolling mobile phone, which no one can live without in today's era, become unmanageable without a low vision aid. Of course, low vision aids in various forms can be found; however, they might not fully satisfy you or give you the feeling of fulfillment. There might be a kind of empty feeling, though you can do things almost like normal. I felt that unexplainable emptiness whenever I saw others having a better perspective because they see things better than me and do things that I miss now. I can't say how it would have felt if I had my other eye in good condition. As the saying goes, "the show must go on", so whatever difficulties and life's challenges we are put into, we must not give up so easily without a fight. Most of life's battles are worth fighting for; the hunger to live is far stronger than anything.

My vision has gone down, but not my hopes. The hunger to live and face whatever life brings. I can say now that I have understood how I need to look into my life now. I understand what better prospects I can expect and can still live life with a harsh eye condition.

One has to understand and properly evaluate the changes this Retinal thing might bring. Disappointment might knock at the door, but that's how life is, and that's what it is. There can't be sunshine every day so keep your Umbrella ready.

There is no denying the fact that whatever I had expressed might not be true with your condition. All that is mentioned at night does not align with your circumstance because on my side here I had visualized most of the happenings concerning Retinal detachment, considering my own experience. I sometimes felt as if I was born with such a curse or paying the penance for the sin of my parents and my forefathers. I was not dealing with any life-threatening condition like cancer, HIV, or whatever, it's a Retinal detachment, in the worst scenario, I could have gone blind or else. I am alive, I should be grateful for the second chance I have, though I fall in the category of partially blind now. The second half of my life could have gone in total blindness; I was lucky I would say so, I have to find a better perspective and an opportunity to do better, even if the road seems doubtful. If somebody asks me how my vision is? My inner voice could be weird and bad now; however, the reality is that any small improvement would be a milestone for me under the given condition. I have follow-up check-ups every three to six months, and I had to go for it for a better perspective. It will not change anything much, but it will protect my eye from any further probable damage. The future might not change much, or my destiny will write a new chapter for my eye condition, perhaps it will help me to survive the uncertainties of life's events for more years to come. I do things considering the boundaries and limitations set due to my eye condition, and sometimes I am heartbroken for it; however, I try to find fulfillment in things I can do. The dream of owning an Aston Martin and driving it might not be a reality; I can drive two-wheelers happily.

The shortcomings that I have after retinal detachment aren't going to change, and I don't expect any miracles like the pastors do. Well, I understand that I can manage most of the basic things and I think that's enough to live the rest of my life. I am not sounding pessimistic here but that's practicality, the reality of my situation.

Your takeaways-

1.   Recovery Period and Restrictions:

Manage your routine life for some time because post-vitrectomy recovery usually takes 2-4 weeks but may extend to months before noticeable vision improvement or in some complicated conditions.

Activities requiring significant eye effort, heavy-duty work, air travel, and weightlifting are restricted, especially if a gas bubble or silicone oil is implanted so don't argue with it and don't try foolish things.

2.   Slow Vision Recovery:

Vision recovery can be slow and sometimes frustrating, particularly with the use of implants like gas bubbles or silicone oil. So, don't be heartbroken, it will take time, so have patience.

Challenges in Daily Life:

Tasks like reading or using mobile phones may require low-vision aids, which might not fully compensate for vision loss, leaving an emotional void.

Emotional Impact:

Feelings of emptiness and comparisons with others having better vision can be disheartening. Try to develop a deeper understanding of life's circumstances and resilience.

3.   Positive Outlook:

Despite vision loss, maintaining hope and adapting to life's challenges with a positive outlook are needed.

4.   Acceptance and Adaptation:

Developing an understanding and evaluating life changes due to retinal detachment helps in managing expectations.

Disappointments are part of life, but resilience and preparedness (symbolized by an umbrella) are crucial.

5.   Gratitude for Life:

Recognizing that partial blindness is not as severe as life-threatening conditions fosters gratitude. Be grateful and find fulfillment within limitations.

6.   Realistic Perspective:

Acceptance of limitations and find joy in manageable activities.

Medical Follow-Ups:

Regular check-ups are necessary to prevent further damage and ensure eye health stability.

7.   Practical Approach to Life:

There are no expectations of miracles but focusing on managing life within the constraints of the condition.

Finding contentment and joy in handling basic life tasks despite limitations.

"Life has other better problems to deal with, I can't stick around with only one problem"- that's what I usually tell myself whenever I feel like it's going above my head. I never thought that handling situations demanded a mature outlook on life, and perhaps this single episode in my life has drawn me to understand life more closely and seriously. It has taught me not to take all goodness in life for granted, but it also never meant to live life in fear and dubious thoughts. There might be an event in life that might happen unexpectedly without your slightest impression and if it happens, have the dauntlessness and willingness to face it, even if it might push you to a situation where you might have to reevaluate your life from scratch, don't lose hope and willingness to live, just not surviving, be a sanguine.

It might sound silly trying to say the same things once again on one another page however I'll do it anyway so saying this, I have tried to put the words in the right order as much as possible trying not to sound too self-centred and tried to justify my current situation after a successful Vitrectomy, whatever happens, happens for a reason. Perhaps if I hadn't faced this circumstance in my life then I might not have ever thought of writing about it in the form of a book in the first place. Writing a book was never on my plate but in the face of the current situation I needed to bring out those barren thoughts that I expected to tell somebody. My story might not be inspiring or can do something in your life on a magnitude scale but I assume that it will rather encourage me to pursue the path that I have chosen so late in the face of life to go. My workability has been impacted a lot; I am not in a position to weep about it but to accept it the way it is now. I have forgiven myself for being so naïve and being somber. I have understood that it will be unfair if I do not discard the thought that my parents did nothing for the sake of my eye. I felt ashamed that at the time I hated them. I might not be able to go back to a 9 to 5 work culture ironically which I miss a lot sometimes.

I will try to find solace in turbulence and I would look up to it without a dubious feeling because I have to go on for the sake of my daughter, for my family, and myself in the end. I have made a few changes in my life prioritizing good health not only physically but mentally too. I don't let any dubious thoughts interfere with my things in life and try to stay positive as much as possible. I do know that I will be heartbroken sometimes but realizing the fact that Life might not change but I need to make changes in the way I look at my life currently.

I may not understand fully someone who has to go through a tough time in life but I do believe that he or she would have the strength and mindset to overcome it someday. We all have our battles to fight, we have to be self-aware of ourselves and expect no guru from the Himalayas would bring the magic salt.

I would be most grateful if I could hear from you. Write to me at dickyd2025@gmail.com.

And one Favor, please, if you could put your valuable thoughts and review for my book, it will help my journey to continue with confidence.

In my recent eye check-up, I got to know that a pre-existing scar is there however it has not interfered with my eye-vision currently.

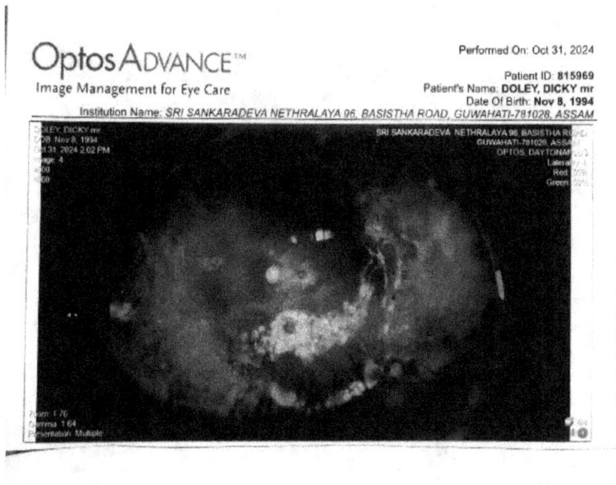

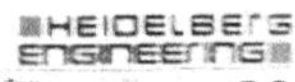

Patient:
Patient ID:
Diagnosis:

DOB:
Exam:
Comment:

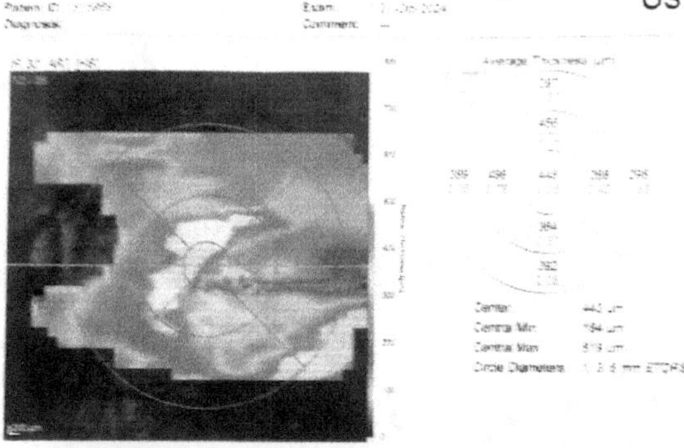

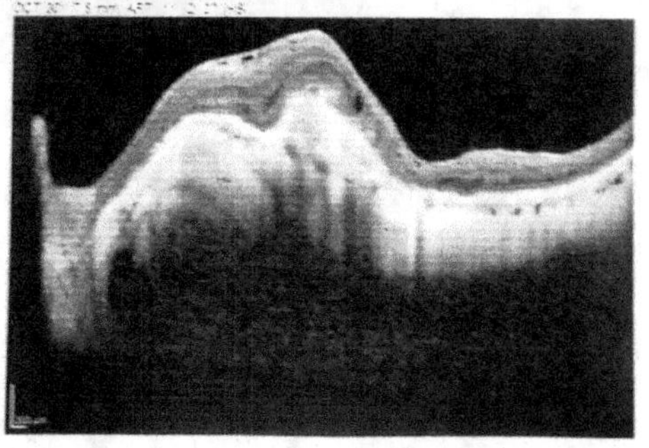

Notes:

Date: 31-10-2024   Signature